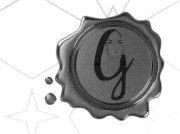

GODDESS
on the GO

RITUALS TO HELP YOU SLOW
DOWN AND *SLAY*

✳

LEORA EDUT

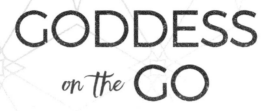

GODDESS
on the GO

Credits

EDITOR: Lisa M. Sundry, www.dragonladyediting.com

DESIGN BY: LeAnna Weller Smith, www.wellersmithdesign.com

ISBN-13: 978-0-692-11465-0

DEDICATION

I dedicate this book to my daughter, Cariel Edut-Daniels. Little do you know, but you are the reason this book was completed. After having a disappointing run with a book agent and several publishing houses, I had given up. I was told that people weren't ready for a collaborative book. And yet, a little less than a year later, you appeared in my belly. I could feel your strength, and then I found out you were an Aries!

I was carrying the strongest person I knew inside of me. From within your personal paradise (a.k.a. my womb), you swirled my body with ideas and inspirations at a time when I thought I would be past exhaustion. One day I was laying on the couch finishing a meditation when I clearly heard you say, "Mama, you must finish the book!" You began exercising your fiery powers and I listened in.

I am so grateful you didn't let me quit on myself. Three years later, you continue to inspire me to do things that scare me and take me places I would never have thought to go.

CONTENTS

INTRODUCTION

SISTERHOOD SAVED MY LIFE

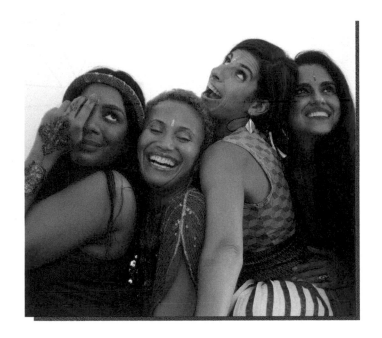

SISTERHOOD SAVED MY LIFE! When I was a young girl, I sauntered around with a luminescent twinkle in my eye. I knew I had bright, shiny magic running through my body! People I met would begin sharing their life stories within five minutes of us meeting. That, to me, was sacred...precious. I knew to treat this with reverence. It was a blessing that others felt seen and safe in this energetic space. Call it the mystical workings of an old soul. These numinous gifts would eventually be needed for something greater.

As I began to move through the harshness of my childhood, I was introduced to mental and physical abuse, rape (as a young adult), and accepting the way society devalued women and girls. A heavy weight of doubt set in as my self-worth began to diminish. Slowly, I bottled up the best parts of me.

I WONDERED: WAS IT NO LONGER OKAY TO BE ALL OF ME ?

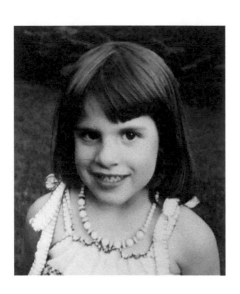

I was four years old the first time I experienced a heartbreaking dose of physical abuse. I can remember the moment clearly, etched forever in my memory, like an invisible scar. Looking back, after years of healing, what impacted me the most was the gaping hole of sadness I felt afterwards. I no longer felt safe and protected. A belief formed that I was unlovable. The people who I thought were heavily invested in my security didn't seem to exist. I had no idea this was tied in to my self-expression, my vivaciousness, which I began to bury. "Was it no longer okay to be *all* of me?" I wondered. Where was that radiant, fearless, big-hearted little girl going? I began to leave my body.

At seven years old, by the grace of Goddess, I was introduced to the Girl Scouts. These ladies had no idea, but they were my answered prayers in the midst of feeling extreme sadness and confusion. Each week I anticipated our meeting. It was there where I was filled with the love and acceptance I so desperately craved. My 7-year-old brain had no clue that I was receiving much-needed deep healing through our emerging sisterhood! It was in their company I could be loud, outrageous, and unafraid. I could be all of *Leora* without the dreaded repercussions at home. The many layers of emotions we inherently carry as women were welcomed in.

The majority of us stayed in this glorious bond of sisterhood until we were 13. Up until this point, nothing could penetrate the power of our bond. However, the numbing pressure of society fell upon each of us—telling us what teenagers "were supposed to do and not do." Suddenly we shut off the voice of our wise inner *guidesses* and fell victim to doing only what "looked cool" to others.

Nothing about being a Girl Scout at age 13 was "acceptable" by our peers. We allowed what others thought was right for us to break up our sacred chain. Our voices suddenly felt squashed! We had allowed society to fuck up the connection that had kept my trust in life going. It was at that time my heart sank—I was losing my most precious asset—sisterhood.

THIS RELATIONSHIP WENT ON AND OFF UNTIL I WAS 19, WHEN HE WAS ARRESTED FOR MURDER. (NOT MINE, THANK GOODNESS.)

Like swinging doors, I was in and out of therapy from ages seven to fifteen. Conveniently, a male doctor prescribed Ritalin to subdue my exuberant self expression, which they diagnosed as "hyperactivity." No one questioned or seemed to care where these unexpected outbursts were coming from. No school counselors showed up at my home, no teachers pried a little deeper. Oh no! Just a "quick, fix it" pill to solve the problem—encouraging the cycle of repressing dark and confusing emotions for a seven-year-old girl who had no idea how to handle what was coming at her.

At age 15, I got into my first romantic relationship. I pictured a tender, loving partner who would cherish having me in his life. He would sweep me off my feet and rescue me from my sadness. I played the story over and over in my head. It would be my golden ticket to the life I always dreamed of!

Obsessively fantasizing, quite the opposite happened. This supposed hero was like a grizzly bear dressed in a puppy

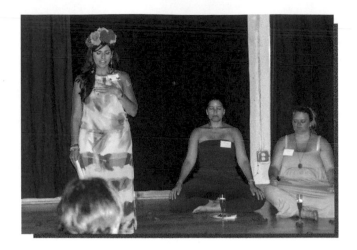

costume. In the beginning he was attentive, adoring, and extremely charismatic. But once the honeymoon period ended, his true colors came out. I felt as if I had to walk on eggshells around him, never knowing if I would be slapped down, cursed at, or stalked. I feared that I had lost the freedom I had once taken for granted in this relationship.

Inside my body, I could feel myself holding onto the trauma and stress I had experienced in childhood. I felt helpless to change any part of that situation. I mean, how does a 15-year-old growing up in the 90's even know where to turn for support? Here I was, this pissed off teenage girl who felt starved for love—and was willing to settle for crumbs. My desperation was evident to every man I came across. I longed to feel deserving and worthy of having love, barely having experienced that from a father who had no parents to show HIM how to express his own love. The cycle of abuse was repeating itself, and I had no idea how to stop it.

I found myself slipping into a bottomless, dark depression. My boyfriend would consistently threaten me with "what would happen" if I left him or, alternately, the way he would hurt himself if I ended the relationship. I walked around life feeling out of control, and I used food as a way to numb out the pain. Every day I walked around judging myself for the situation I was in. It seemed I couldn't find a way out. NO ONE knew about the abuse, as I felt so much shame for allowing this to happen to me! Between the self-judgment and holding onto this dark secret, I fell deeper into despair.

This tumultuous relationship went on and off until I was 19, when he was arrested for murder. (Not mine, thank goodness.) My self-worth began to return a little more each day after this. Divine intervention at its finest! I made a promise to a higher power above that I would NEVER, EVER let another man put his hands on me without telling someone about what was happening. I attempted to hide my scars of grief and rage. Not really doing a good job of that, I turned to food and alcohol to ease the pain, when it was too much to bear.

Along came the next Prince Charming, this one promising me wealth and love. He was running fake insurance jobs out of his repair garage and he convinced me to partake in the hustle. Being deeply attached to finding that someone who was going to love me and save me from myself, I was willing to do anything!

One morning, I was doing my client's nails in my parent's basement when there was a knock at the back door. The Feds! (Apparently, Prince Charming was running the scam on a large scale with his entire family, and they were all being watched.) I was facing the possibility of spending 10 years in prison. Lawyers got involved, and if it weren't for having a pristine record, I could have ended up losing out on a large chunk of life behind bars.

It became my norm to spend the majority of my time intoxicated. I'd find half days wasted on romanticizing. Evening after evening, you could find me in the hottest club in Detroit—drinking champagne and longing for approval from the opposite sex. This is what I had thought was "luxurious living."

After several hours of bubbly into the wee hours of night, I would lose sight of any clear judgement. Often I woke up with killer hangovers, having fallen for men who had numerous red flags over their foreheads that I ignored.

Sex was the way I used my body to feel any ounce of emotion. I had shut down, protecting myself from the fear of feeling any pain. Over and over again, I attracted unconscious men who picked up on my desperation and low self-esteem. They would take me out for drinks, which would usually end in date rape. I found myself in a vicious cycle of waking up in a drunken daze, questioning my choices. This cycle reflected all of my suppressed self-hate and insecurities.

DURING ONE OF THOSE SLEEPLESS NIGHTS, MY FEMININE INTUITION BUSTED DOWN MY RESISTANCE. I HEARD A VOICE THAT CAME THROUGH SO CLEARLY: LEORA, YOU CAN'T STAY HERE ANYMORE.

"T" came into my life a year and a half before I moved to NYC. He was a contrast to all the other guys of my past. T reminded me of a huge *teddy* bear. He treated me with a loving kindness I had longed for, was extremely generous in all the ways I needed, and let me see his sensitive side. On the flip side of the coin, he was a huge drug dealer who, after being robbed, slept with guns by his bed.

At 24, I started playing with the reality of my future. Was I going to find myself caught in the middle of a drug shoot out, or do time for being his girlfriend? These paralyzing thoughts kept me up into the wee hours of night. I had formed a habit of pushing away my feelings and invalidating my truth.

During one of those sleepless nights, my feminine intuition was able to move past my resistance. I heard a voice that came through so clearly: *Leora, you can't stay here anymore.*

Like everything that is in divine order, my mother called me out of the blue to have a chat about "What my life's goals were." Looking back, I can see that my mom had tapped into her own divine insight in that moment, her radar sensing that "something was off" in her daughter's life.

As we spoke, I could feel a sadness rising up in my chest. There was a heaviness in my belly and heart. I believed I was a failure and that my family thought this, too. I had NO idea what I truly wanted to do in my life; there was no connection to any source of passion. Where would I find the answers to these questions? *I was so blocked off from my intuition.* I latched onto my mom's solution of applying to fashion school and moving to New York, feeling a desperate call for change. Anything sounded more appealing than my dead-end current circumstances.

The application for school arrived, but my self-confidence was shattered into pieces. I didn't feel worthy of filling one word out. Somewhere along the way, I had formed a voice in my mind that said I was stupid. Who the hell did I think I was, attending a prestigious school in NYC? Who in the fuck was I fooling? I wasn't really going anywhere. And how could I leave T? Or my faithful nail clients who had traveled with me from salon to salon? And what about my current circle of friends *du jour*, who I popped champagne with on the regular? Surely, they'd all be devastated if I left!

My mother was going to battle against my deepest fear of not being *good enough*. Each week she would call to find out if I had filled out my application for FIT. Procrastination mixed with terror responded: "Next week, Mom." I had no idea how to let go of the "control" I thought I had over my life and step into TRUST. The fear I felt paralyzed me from making any forward movement. This was combined with the worst possible thoughts of how my life was going to turn out.

BUT THE JOY COULD NOT FULLY SETTLE IN AS MY REALITY FELT LIKE A MIXED BAG OF HOLY FUCKS.

I was six months into this cycle of driving myself cray cray, putting off my FIT application, when the holy spirit kicked in! One day I woke up, sat down at the computer table and began typing, putting my heart and soul into that essay. The hairs on my arms stood up. I could feel my heart beat. A sense of re-aliveness was kicking in!

Once submitted, waiting on a response to that application was one of the big tests from Life. Like when you lose 50 pounds and someone invites you to your favorite buffet with all the luscious desserts you still dream about, or *that* ex reaches out with an enticing text message—the one who you have zero willpower to resist—you feel the overwhelming pressure to fucking fold like a deck of tarot cards.

For me, it was being caught up in a lifestyle that was glamorously dangerous. Unfortunately, I failed this particular Life Test, when one day a girlfriend convinced me to put some extra things in a bag at a high-end mall in Detroit. Instead of trusting my inner voice that was shouting, "Hell, NO! Been there, done that!" I gave in to her consistent pressure. Sure enough, one month later I was facing a 10-year prison sentence. It felt as if I was on a roller coaster of self-sabotage and there was no getting off.

Six months later, when that crisp, white envelope with the black "FIT" logo finally arrived in my mailbox, I was caught in a combination of extreme doubt and a desire for a miracle. *What if this IS for me?* My hands shaking, I carefully opened the letter. There it was, on that page: "Leora Edut, you have been accepted to The Fashion Institute of Technology of New York City." I had to read it 10 more times before it sank in—I was accepted, and holy shit, I was moving to the Big Apple!! The first person I called was my mom, screaming with excitement.

But the joy could not fully settle in as my reality felt like a mixed bag of holy fucks. I had an upcoming trial for that shoplifting case with one of the toughest judges in Oakland county. I had kept this secret from my parents and most people, feeling overwhelmed by the repercussions I was possibly facing. Leading up to the trial, my days were consumed with terror. I could be locked up for a year without my family knowing what had happened or how to reach me.

I could feel hard knots in my belly as I walked into the courthouse that early Friday morning. Had I just thrown my NYC school future away? When they called my name, my attorney confidently presented the FIT college acceptance letter to the judge. In that moment my heart dropped down to my feet. I was in complete panic—my body tensed up—ready to receive the worst news.

But the angels above had another plan for me. It was as if I was watching a movie play out before my eyes. The judge's stern face softened. She turned to me and asked if I was looking forward to going away to school. I answered "YES!" without hesitating.

My grandmother's spirit had to be in the room that day, as I was sentenced to only six months' probation!

Spirit spoke through me again as I was driving home: "Don't worry about figuring things out with T, you're going to New York!"

THAT SAYING, 'EVERYWHERE YOU GO, THERE YOU ARE,' WAS MY NEVER-ENDING STORY.

Quietly, I began making my plans to move to NYC, telling a few of my manicurist clients and friends. I flew down to New York to find my new home. With my sister's help, we found my new tiny studio apartment on West End and 71st in one day. My angels were by my side as I made this new transition.

Leora, the girl who believed the dark reality of her life was something she couldn't escape. The one who felt defeated by life, and certainly didn't think she was good enough to go to any fancy NYC school, was moving 614.34 miles across the country. OMYGODDESS!

I arrived in NYC with this unrealistic expectation that everything would effortlessly fall in my lap. T was going to stop selling drugs and move out to NYC with me, numerous jobs were going to gracefully line up, and I would have this fabulous, supportive group of friends. Life would be perfect now that I had left my past behind in Detroit!

At least, that's what I continued telling myself. That saying, "Everywhere you go, there you are," was my truth. The way I felt about myself on the inside remained full of panic and uncertainty. NYC was welcoming me in with a proper giant ass kicking. T wasn't up for changing his ways or moving to NYC. The waitressing job interview at a very sought after restaurant—which I "knew" I had in the bag—turned into a horrendous nightmare when I couldn't open up a bottle of wine. And I hadn't made a single friend!

Tears streamed down my face that evening as I left the interview and walked down 72nd street. I had $7 left to my name and no clue as to where the next source of income was coming from. Feeling as if I had no friends to turn to, I called my mother, who reminded me I wasn't alone out there. Shame and guilt ran through my body. I felt like such a fraud living in NYC. What had I talked myself into? Leaving my comfort zone in Detroit, where I had made it, for this? As I continued sitting in my sadness, that feeling of rock bottom hit me.

When the first guy I met in NYC wanted me to participate in a credit card scam, it hit me that I *may* have a role in attracting the same situation, even though I told myself I had changed. I felt desperate for something new but I had no idea where to turn.

WHY IS EVERYONE FREAKIN? SMILING? WHO DRANK THE KOOL–AID?! HOLY SHIT!

DIVINE INTERVENTION HAD NOW BECOME A PATTERN IN MY LIFE THAT I COULDN'T QUITE SEE YET. My sisters had spoken about some sort of transformational work they were doing. In 2002, spiritual work was far from mainstream. To most people I knew, that shit seemed way too "weird."

Back then people weren't all excited to take an honest look at themselves. I had no clue what "spiritual work" meant—or what I was signing myself up for. But what I couldn't deny was that my introverted older sisters, who I had known my entire life, had become these confident, self-expressed women who were unashamed to go after their biggest dreams. From getting a book deal with Simon & Schuster to becoming the official astrologers for Teen People Magazine, well, let's just say I desired for some of THAT to rub off on me!

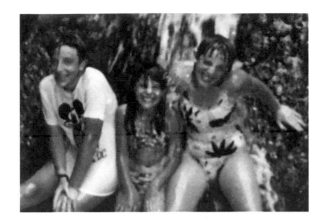

My sister invited me to an intro night to check out the "work" she had been doing. I had attended one of these events a few months earlier with my mom, but this time I was ready to listen. This time, I had a whole new level of humility and openness that I did not have before. My prior attitude was, "Why is everyone freakin' smiling? Who drank the Kool-Aid?! Holy SHIT!" It felt weird!

Fast forward, and I'm back in that same building, dragging my feet. There was a ripple of excitement, where I could feel the hairs stand up on the back of my neck, coupled with an apprehension in my belly. What was I really going to get from spending a weekend in a room? I mean, was a weekend REALLY gonna change my life?

The second time around WAS completely different, and so many of the things the woman who was speaking overcame resonated with me. She was standing up on stage, proud of her past, owning it with such power, and she had created a brilliant life for herself.

Yes, sign ME up!

By Sunday, I had released a heavy weight of guilt and shame that I had been carrying everywhere I went. No longer did I feel like a victim because of my past. It was as if I had set myself free and there was an opening to reinvent my life in this moment.

I made peace with my father. Something I definitely could never have seen coming. In my gut, I knew there was more to explore.

This was the beginning of something new. I was going to get to know and love *Leora*. For the first time in many years, I was able to feel my emotions.

I devoured everything I could learn about—discovering the yummy art of romantic relationships, effective communication between women and men, and an empowered way to look at my finances. I became a master at producing results.

MY LIFE WAS A CONTRADICTION OF SPENDING WEEKENDS IN SEMINARS, HELPING OTHER PEOPLE CONNECT WITH THEIR PASSIONS, WHILE WATCHING THE DAYS PASS BY AND DOING NOTHING ABOUT MY OWN.

Results became an addiction for me! I used them as validation that I was worthy. My ego needed a way to prove that I was better than others, and to convince myself that—spiritually—I was evolving.

And yet...there was an unsatisfied feeling that met me every

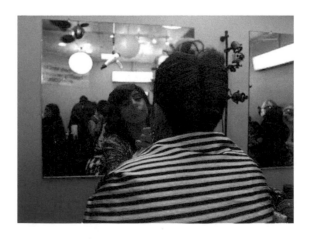

morning when I woke up and every evening when I lay my head down to rest. *What the fuck was it?* I couldn't quite place my finger on it. Wasn't I doing the work? *What the hell was wrong with me?*

As time went on, my life had become a contradiction of spending weekends in seminars, helping other people connect with their passions, while watching the days pass by and doing nothing about my own. I would come home and isolate myself in my apartment, stuffing down my intuition with rich vegan desserts.

The deeper connection to my feminine power was desperately missing—and I had no idea. At 26, I had become a celebrity makeup artist, and my job was to climb the star status ladder. It didn't matter if I had to compete with so-called "friends" to get the job, or hang out till the wee hours taking tequila shots, ignoring the needs of my own body for rest and self-care. But regardless of the amount of "work" I did, I became the infamous mouse chasing the cheese. I was desperately clawing for romantic love, yet consistently dating men for periods of time who couldn't commit. My financial state was either feast or famine.

I WOULD COME HOME AND ISOLATE MYSELF IN MY APARTMENT, STUFFING DOWN MY INTUITION WITH RICH VEGAN DESSERTS.

Balance was a seven-letter word that I had never learned, and I found myself in a pattern of habitually over-giving. Something was off here! Wasn't I doing all this transformational stuff to trust that there was *enough* in the world, to empower others around me, and to have an amazing life that would want to make me pinch myself every morning?

I STOPPED QUESTIONING WHERE MY LIFE WAS GOING AND SANK INTO THE ENERGY OF BEING HELD, LOVED UP, BY THESE OTHER WOMEN.

In 2012, that thing that I could feel so deeply in my body that was missing was revealed. It was, simply, sisterhood. SISTERHOOD—that same glorious energy that had taken me through the darkness of my childhood was, finally, rediscovered.

It was reinvented in my small one bedroom apartment on 34th Street, and was inspired by my biological sisters, who were headed off to do a course on...SISTERHOOD.

Hearing that word brought chills to every part of my body. I was curious and excited to experience real friendships with other women. I invited seven women (who normally wouldn't have chosen each other as friends) to be a part of this goddess circle. All seven of them said, "YES!" This was my first indication that women yearn to come out of isolation and be in communities where they feel visible to other women. In so many parts of the world women long to have a place to share their truth and be vulnerable and yet have no idea where to go.

Trusting other women was one of the biggest challenges I faced in the beginning of sisterhood. I was so used to competing with other women and putting other women down to make myself look better. In that vicious cycle, I had found myself alternating between being the mean girl and *being* "mean-girled." I had learned to protect my feelings. There were fears of being judged for being "too much" or "not enough"; for not having the "picture perfect" life behind closed doors. What a number the patriarchy does to women who are searching to live their best lives. Somehow, we can't find our power in this shit show of ways we are taught to idealize ourselves as women. No wonder I was drawn to something that felt like the complete opposite.

As each new week went by, I witnessed my stories being held as precious, sacred. No one was trash talking about another sister behind her back. I stopped questioning where my life was going and sank into the energy of being held, loved up, by these other women. Life was getting GOOD as I followed my mouthwatering desires. I was done making shit harder for myself than it had to be. I continued to unpeel and reveal layers of myself: As each one was out there for everyone to see in our circle, instead of it being pulled apart and analyzed, it was celebrated, and honored for its beauty!

What happened next was even more lavish! I got a whiff of:
The tantalizing spell that women of the world can turn on and off;
The essence that lives inside of every woman; and
The deep love and care we share with one another that can heal
wounds for which we think there is no cure.

I had found the buried treasure that had been missing in my life, and in the lives of most women I knew.

COLLECTIVELY, WE STARTED CALLING IN WHAT WE HAD BEEN DREAMING ABOUT FOR YEARS—AND HAD DONE YEARS OF TRANSFORMATIONAL WORK AND THERAPY FOR!

After two years of meeting every week, each one of our lives looked completely different than when we began. Collectively, we started calling in what we had been dreaming about for years—and had done years of transformational work and therapy for! It was FUN! It was full of joy, ease—and having the support of sisterhood in the roughest of moments or facing our deepest fears was like soaking in a rose gold bath.

SISTERHOOD IS THE HIDDEN MEDICINE BAG FOR ALL WOMEN. MOST OF THE TIME YOU DON'T EVEN KNOW YOU NEED IT.

One day things became crystal clear. My truth was revealed, which was to bring sisterhood forth into the world. To help as many women in the world experience what they had no idea they had been missing out on, too.

Sisterhood is the hidden medicine bag for all women. Most of the time you don't even know you need it. When you allow it in, everything in your life shifts from your cellular makeup to the way your life looks on the outside. Shame and guilt no longer have a VIP seat at your dinner table. Loneliness gets a firm ass kicking out your front door! You no longer obsess over your body, as you begin to admire your breathtaking curves and notice that, as you give approval, others do, too. You give the middle finger to unhealthy relationships, mediocre living, or putting up with your circumstances. You become a grand reflection of the way your sisters see you—AS A GODDESS!

It's an indescribable feeling to be in relationships with women where you experience a flow—where you are receiving first, and then giving from a place of fullness. Your thirst for life is BACK! You are ready to claim your succulence, call in your luscious desires, and reawaken your birthright to experiencing an abundance-filled life, and you design that life on your own terms! It's time for you to experience all of this, and so much more.

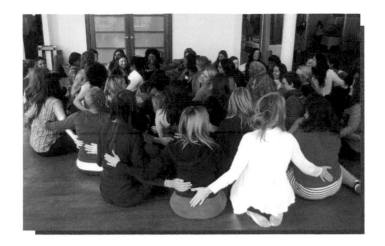

As you turn each page of this book, you will be guided by some of the women who have made a profound impact on my life. The rituals and exercises they share with you have been my go-to's when I have swum the depths of my darkest nights of the soul. My wish is that you will read this book with your closest girlfriends, in book clubs, at your job, on the subway/airplanes, and share your experiences together in sacred sisterhood! ✳

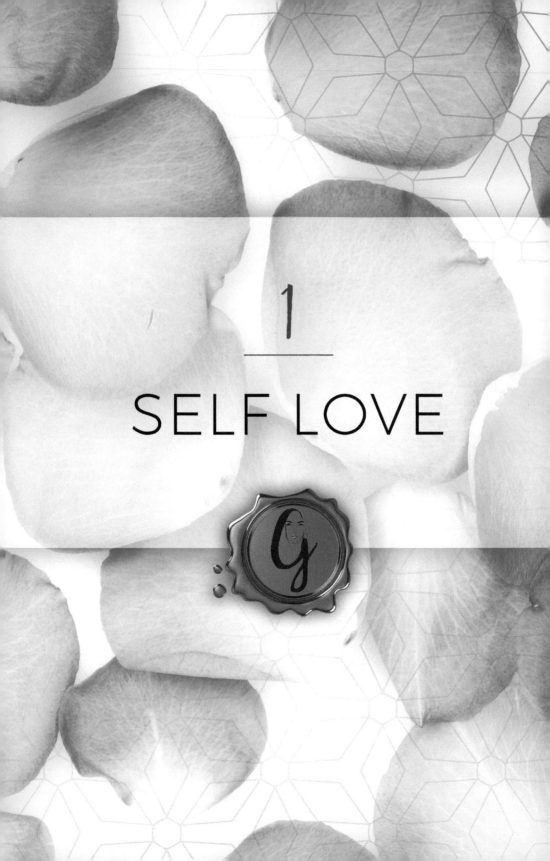

1

SELF LOVE

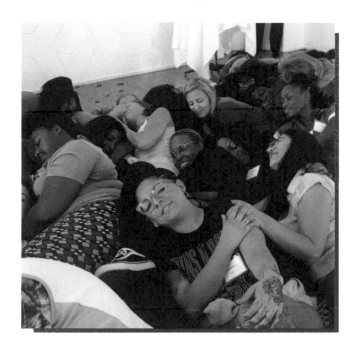

A

T AGE 32, I HAD JUST BEGUN TO LEARN ABOUT SELF-LOVE. It baffles me that this is not thought of as important to teach in school as math and science! It would have saved me years of body hating, shame, and binge eating. For decades I looked outside of myself for validation that I was loved. I thought a part of "loving myself" was eating decadent food and dating lots of men I didn't really care about, while pretending to have the time of my life. Isn't that what society paints as the picture of what the "ideal" woman wants? There had been no lessons in honoring myself. I had no idea how to worship my body with love and compassion. Or that I could discover pleasure by the simple act of inhaling a gorgeous bouquet of flowers!

It was time to reconnect to the feelings deep in my well that had been suppressed by a masculine-dominated society.

And so it began in my own tiny one bedroom apartment on 34th street that seven women got together each week to re-welcome in our divine truth: It was time for us to repossess the power that we had given away, to see ourselves as precious, golden vessels that came from a powerful lineage. We could no longer hide or ignore that. It was time to let go of our inner "mean girl."

SELF–CARE BEGAN WITH FIVE MINUTES OF MEDITATION WITHOUT CHECKING MY PHONE.

Self-love meant making choices that put me at the forefront and no longer at the back; it was choosing to be around women who would hold me through my tears AND grab my hands and dance wildly in the streets for our own pleasure!

I began to feel safe to open up and be vulnerable around my goddess sisters, sharing things that in the past would have made me cringe, that I would have held inside out of fear of looking bad. Things like, "I am not happy with the way my body feels and looks," and, "I don't know how I'm going to pay my rent this month!" Shit was really REAL in the sisterhood and, for the first time, just saying those things out loud gave me freedom. I had been carrying so much shame, walking around in life telling myself, "I should have it ALL together by now!" Yet these beautiful sisters held a container for me to unpeel all my layers, get emotionally butt-bootie naked, and they loved me through each one of my imperfections. Through this I began to recreate my life with VIBRANCE, outrageousness, and to own my sensuality that had been put on the shelf.

My walls began to come down—no faster than they were supposed to—but for the first time, I felt alive, loved, and like I finally belonged.

The goddesses held this jewel-encrusted container for me and encouraged me to look at the value I brought into the world. They reflected back to me that I was a force, a bad ass goddess who could say NO to anything that didn't align with that. Suddenly I began to turn down male companions and opportunities that I felt were just not a good use of my time. I learned that "NO" is a complete sentence, and that an explanation was just not necessary anymore. This certainly wasn't easy for someone who had been trained to be a people pleaser.

As I practiced honoring my precious time and savoring my worth, the more AH-MAZING I felt. I was getting to my seductive deep-down-there desires. It felt. . . like a rebirth at 32!

This new self-love practice made sure it acquainted me well with her cousin, self-care. I definitely didn't have time for THAT previously! The masculine part of me had been running the show. My favorite words had always been "I'm busy." I equated that to mean I was "important." Yet my body was suffering. I never felt good or had any energy. My M.O was to focus all my fuel on my business. Life was passing me by without a drip drop of JOY! I often questioned why I was even living in this city—just to pay a NYC rent? There had to be something better!

Self-care began with five minutes of meditation without checking my phone. I was so worried that I would be *missing out* on some important text or email! I had no idea that I AM my body; I became aware that—NO—my life did not fall apart from five extra minutes with Deepak, and so I began to push my edge.

SELF–LOVE IS ALL ABOUT CONSISTENT PRACTICE AND NEVER ABOUT PERFECTION.

As I began to embody this "goddess thing" as a full-fledged lifestyle that I wasn't going to part with, life started to get really yummy. This self-love protocol began to feel like the life I had always desired! And so I shimmied and hip circled before business calls instead of stressing the fuck out. Days were filled with rich conversations with my goddess sisters, instead of running back and forth to the fridge. I received consistent energy healings to work through built up anxiety, instead of spending hours self-analyzing what was wrong with me.

SELF-LOVE IS ABOUT THE PRACTICE AND NEVER ABOUT PERFECTION. If you're reading this book, I'm sure you already have a full life, and you may even have some rituals in your goddess tool bag, but let's be 100% honest with ourselves: Sometimes those tools get old and crusty. At times we may need a little fire lit up under our asses . . . a gentle nudging or reminder that our bodies are feeling worn to the bone and *restless* because they need some extra loving care. How about some succulent tools to feel re-inspired about life? Or just the time and space to be alone with our darkness?

I want to support that appetite of yours that wants to taste how brilliant and delectable your life can get—in a "make-you-wanna-shake-your-ass-all-day" kind of flow!

In the next few pages, you get to immerse yourself in a pool of JUICE-A-LICIOUS rituals from some of my absolute favorite fellow goddesses that will remind you (and everyone you know) that the HAWT, all-powerful, ab-fab Goddess that is you is BACK! ✳

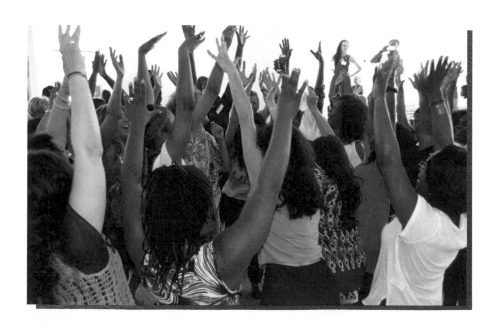

"

THIS SELF-LOVE PROTOCOL BEGAN TO FEEL LIKE THE LIFE I HAD ALWAYS DESIRED! AND SO I SHIMMIED AND HIP CIRCLED BEFORE BUSINESS CALLS INSTEAD OF STRESSING THE FUCK OUT.

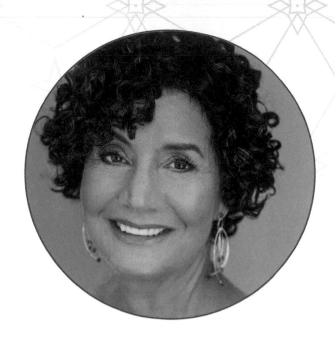

Self Love

———

ESSENTIAL OILS~ESSENTIAL SELF

✳

Divinely Contributed by

VALERIE BENNIS

Introduction

IN 2008, WHEN WE WERE ALL BEING FORCE-
FED BY THE MEDIA TO *DO MORE, BE MORE,*
self-care was frowned upon, viewed as frivolous girlie stuff. (Toughen up, women. Don't you dare go thinking about yourself!) In the midst of this patriarchal mindset, there was one goddess I became aware of who chose to follow the essence of her own truth. The goddess I'm referring to is Valerie Bennis, or as we call her—Vali. I was mesmerized by the way she moved through the room with a soft calmness and confidence. It was unlike anything I had ever seen. It wasn't bold or loud, yet you could feel it the moment you laid eyes on her. I was intimidated by the level of feminine energy she displayed, I had never experienced such power.

One day, I mustered the courage to approach her. We got into a conversation about the body and how important it is to listen to its needs. Vali spoke with me about weeklong, luxe self-care retreats she attended. She shared how she had learned to slow down and tune in to the messages her body was sending her. Whether that was to rest, eat healthy, move her body in ways that felt good, or retreat in nature for some self-care pampering. This goddess was painting a picture of a life I desired to have a taste of!

Following her lead, I began by waking up my body with magnificent nourishment and care. Through yummy massages, daily meditation and delicious feminine movement classes, a sense of aliveness and gratitude returned to my life. My inner guidess gave me the double wink, hi-five, and hip circle indicating that choosing pleasure over obligation, and honoring my feelings, was the true path towards my self-love.

THE SENSE OF SMELL AND TOUCH ARE AWAKENED WITH THE AROMAS OF NATURE AND THE FEEL OF JOJOBA AGAINST YOUR SKIN— NOURISHING, SOFTENING, AND LIGHTLY SCENTING YOUR PATH.

When I knew self-love was going to be included in this book, I thought, Who better to take part than Vali, who I consider "The Queen of Self-Love"? Vali's passion is oozing out in every bit of this ritual. She covers the gamut on how to nurture your self-care morning, noon, and night. We will commence this self-love party not with an Amen, but an A-WOMAN! ✳

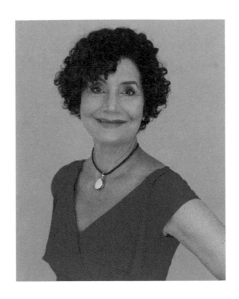

Q&A

WITH VALERIE BENNIS

L: **Why do you believe self-care rituals are becoming non-negotiables for women?**

V: Self-care rituals provide the space to take a "pause" in your busy life. It's a time for yourself, and yourself only. I believe it's important for women to take care of themselves in all aspects—mentally, emotionally, and spiritually. This is one way for a woman to address all of these areas. In our culture there is a lot of pressure for women to look and be a certain way. Often women end up with a bunch of insecurities about how they look and how they are. This is a way for them to stop the inner self-critic and be kind to themselves.

Women also juggle a great deal and are under stress from daily living. Self-care rituals are a way to enjoy "me" time away from all the pressures of daily life. They are known to reconnect us to our sensuality, which as women is an integral part of who we are—of our essential self. Taking part in these rituals is like taking a deep, healing breath.

I THINK SELF–LOVE IS A REQUIREMENT FOR LEADING A HEALTHY AND EMPOWERED LIFE.

L: **Vali is the creator of Essence of Vali. Many of us have heard about the magnitude essential oils can have in helping heal the body. I thought it would be fun to hear some of your personal favorite stories.**

V: One of my clients was the daughter of an elderly man. Her father was having a lot of trouble sleeping due to pain. She and her daughter (his granddaughter) both used the "Relief" massage & bath oil, gently massaging him; and he was able to sleep. Another client who had cancer was calmed by using the "Sleep Bedtime Balm." She dabbed it above her upper lip and experienced immediate relief from her stress and sadness. A third client's mother was hit by a car; she used our mists for comforting during her intense grieving process.

L: **If you were given a shiny bullhorn and could shout out one vital thing about women and self-love what would that be?**

V: I think self-love is a requirement for leading a healthy and empowered life. So many times when we have disappointments and setbacks, our self-esteem suffers and takes a hit. Self-care rituals are a way to bring us back to our most empowered self and put us back in touch with the love that we feel for ourselves.

DAILY ESSENTIAL OIL RITUALS

Essential oils can enhance the daily goddess experience by soothing, inspiring and celebrating one's body, mind and spirit. The sense of smell and touch are awakened with the aromas of nature and the feel of jojoba against your skin—nourishing, softening, and lightly scenting your path.

THE PLEASURE OF BATHING CAN NEVER BE UNDERESTIMATED.

Sensual Start to the Day

Every morning when I arise, I first turn on my diffuser filled with bergamot and orange (very uplifting) and then proceed to dry brush my skin. Brush your bare skin in upward strokes. It is very stimulating and great for exfoliating the skin. Take a massage oil and massage your body, taking time to appreciate the feel of your own skin; knowing that you are honoring your body with this self-care ritual. Spray your face with rose water. Pure rose water is a by-product of the distillation process of rose oil. Top it off with a warm shower.

Mid-Afternoon Practice

A diffuser is something essential to have. You can keep it in your office or wherever you work from. Usually I fill it with uplifting citrus essential oils such as bergamot, orange, lemon, lime and grapefruit. About 3 p.m. is when most people experience a slump in energy. Being a health nut, I rarely eat sugar and never drink coffee and, instead, reach for an uplifting mist and mist the air around myself. Sometimes I apply the mist to my hands and then inhale the aroma directly. Or I use an aromatherapy inhaler. Taking a moment to breathe in an energizing essential oil immediately shifts your energy.

Bedtime Ritual

The pleasure of bathing can never be underestimated. I often think of what it would be like if everyone practiced this ritual at night. First fill your tub, adding a cup of Epsom salts as the water fills the tub. Once the tub is full, add a couple capfuls of a relaxing aromatic bath oil. For up to twenty minutes, enjoy the water surrounding your body and savor the oil against your skin. Take a moment to breathe in the aroma of essential oils and release the cares of the day. Some of my favorite essential oils with sedative properties are: lavender, cedarwood, ylang/ylang, chamomile and marjoram.

Once out of your bath, massage your feet with an aromatic oil, paying attention to your toes and the areas of your feet that need special care. When you get into bed, either mist the pillowcase or put a few drops of a relaxing scented oil (I use the "Bedtime Ritual") on the corner of the pillowcase to relax into a peaceful sleep.

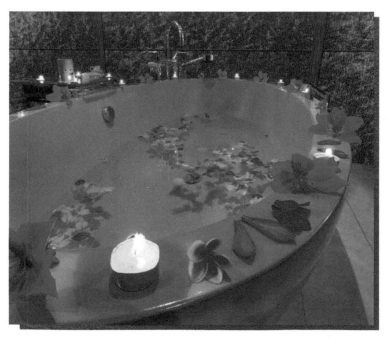

A Love Ritual

Soak in a fragrantly exotic bath with your lover by adding two capfuls of bath oil to a full tub–swirl water with hands to distribute aroma. Enjoy giving and receiving a sensual massage. Mist room, sheets and pillowcases with an aphrodisiac aromatherapy mist to magnify the sensuality of your time together. You can also use as a body mist to increase the level of intensity.

APHRODISIAC ESSENTIAL OILS ARE: Clove, Rosewood, Sweet Orange, Ginger, Patchouli, Ylang/Ylang, Rose, Rosewood and Sandalwood.

ABOUT VALERIE

Valerie Bennis, founder and president of Essence of Vali, is a certified aromatherapist who has won industry awards for her 100% natural formulas. Her mission is for all people to experience the benefits of natural plant essences through the use of her special line of products. The company is known for the beautiful aromas of their proprietary blends, the effectiveness of each formula and their appeal to women, children and men of all ages. Valerie is personally moved and touched by the stories that she hears from people that are benefitting from the products. The mission of the company is to create healing and beauty through plant essences and to demonstrate that natural essences go way beyond simply being "nice smells"–they have powerful healing properties for health and well being.

Visit Valerie at: www.essenceofvali.com ✳

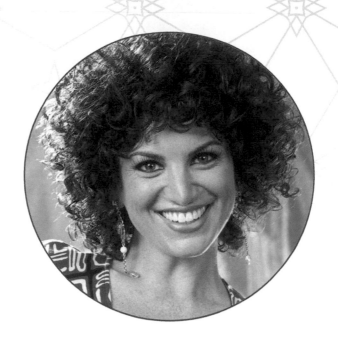

Self Love

"BOOTY PARLOR"

✳

Divinely Contributed by

DANA B. MYERS

Introduction

GET YOUR FANS OUT AND TURN YOUR AC ON, IT'S ABOUT TO GET HAWT IN HERE!

I introduce to you Dana Myers, a goddess who is dripping with sensuality and fucking unapologetic about every drop of it. We met at the beginning of my exploration into the feminine. My body instantly sensed there was something this gorgeous red-headed bombshell of a woman could teach me. As we began to spend time together, I watched Dana in action. She gave me permission to feel the hot steaminess of being turned on, to explore what pleasure feels like in my body. My big "A-Ha!" moment was realizing that flirting was for my OWN enjoyment!

Dana is a mojo connoisseur—I've watched her take a mother of five, who has forgotten she has the power to make her man come-hither, and transform that mamma into a being who knows she is so smoking hot that she creates traffic jams as she strides by! Dana's belief that every goddess merits a daily dose of self-pleasuring is why I knew she had the SKILLZ to give us the low-low on embracing our inner vixens. It's time for us to have zero shame and own the shit out of our raw sexiness and sass! ✳

LOOK INTO YOUR OWN EYES AND TELL YOURSELF HOW MUCH YOU LOVE YOURSELF.

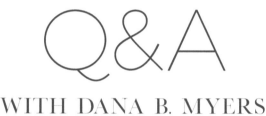

WITH DANA B. MYERS

L: **Why do you think so many women shy away from being in touch with their erotic being?**

D: I believe that sex and sexiness are as important as eating, drinking and working out, and yet, more often than not, so many of us are willing to set our sensuality aside, dismiss its importance, or simply let it drift to the back burner of our busy, multi-tasking daily lives. You get overbooked with your kids' activities and social commitments, and convince yourself that you have "no time" for sex. Or, you get lazy in your long term relationship and forget how much sex matters! For many women in today's hyper-entrepreneurial culture, it's easy to become uber-focused on building your business and forego your passionate side in order to "get things done." Or, perhaps you received negative messages about sex during your childhood and never found the courage or help to work through them and find your free, sensual self.

IF YOU THINK YOU SHINE AT THE OFFICE, MAKE THE WORLD'S BEST WIFE AND MOTHER, OR HAVE A PERSONAL STYLE THAT'S VOGUE–WORTHY, SIMPLY WAIT UNTIL YOUR SENSUALITY IS ON FULL–TILT.

There are so many reasons women shy away from their sensuality, and they're all quite personal and nuanced. However, there's a beautiful movement happening that's encouraging women to embrace and own our sensual sides—and I'm happy to be a part of it!

L: **How are sensuality and self-love like kissing cousins?**

D: When you become the sexiest, most fabulous and vibrant version of you—with full-throttle confidence, self-love, and an active pursuit of the sexual satisfaction you deserve—all of your life's other endeavors will benefit.

You become happier, healthier, calmer, more successful, more whole. I see it time and time again. If you think you shine at the office, make the world's best wife and mother, or have a personal style that's Vogue-worthy, simply wait until your sensuality is on full-tilt. Perhaps most importantly, owning your sensuality naturally encourages you to soften up on yourself. By living a more sensual life—with more sexual satisfaction—

your "perceived flaws" start to become "perfect imperfections" because you've become more aware of your body's ability to receive pleasure. And all this equals deeper, richer, more magnificent self-love!

L: **Would you share with our goddesses one of your favorite client stories where a woman took back her own sexual power?**

D: There are so many stories that've touched my heart, it's hard to pick a favorite! There was the woman who realized that her ability to experience pleasure was far greater than her size—she dropped her shame about what size jeans she wore and started celebrating the size and depth of her orgasms instead! There's the mom who brought her marriage back from the brink of divorce just by following my simple sex schedule for four weeks. She recommitted to intimacy with her husband, and they learned to communicate about sex and sensuality in a whole new way. It was like a rebirth for them! All the stories wow me, because even the smallest of awakenings means I'm doing good work in the world!

Creating Seductive Beauty & Body Rituals

Before you can love sharing your body with a partner of your choosing, first you need to learn how to love that body yourself! I always say that confidence is the sexiest thing you can have, and creating seductive body rituals is one of the most powerful tools you have for buffing up your sexy self-confidence. Here's one ritual that'll give you a chance to flirt with yourself, meditate in the mirror, and have simple, sexy fun all while boosting your body confidence in a major way.

The Ritual: Exploring your assets from the neck down

It's time to focus your attention downward and pay some loving attention to that gorgeous body of yours. This is one ritual that worships the whole neck-to-toe package at once. It's going to require you to let go of your negative body banter and really embrace & adore yourself—just as you are, right now, today.

To start, strip down and stand in front of a full-length mirror. Put on a bra and panties that you love, or better yet, wear nothing at all.

Next, turn on some music. Take some time to delicately caress lotion into your skin. Check yourself out. Give yourself a smile or a wink, or both. Look into your own eyes and tell yourself how much you love yourself.

Then, start complimenting your feminine curves. Give each curve, each part, some loving attention. This may feel strange at first, but I promise you, the more you do this, the more you're going to fall in love with yourself. There are glorious positives about your body and I want you to see them, too. Here's some body part inspiration to get you going with this ritual!

NECK, SHOULDERS AND COLLARBONE. These are universally erogenous parts—a mere whisper of breath on them can get your blood pumping. With a fingertip, trace the curves and contours and take pleasure in the way your smooth, soft skin reacts to your touch. Say something lovely to yourself.

BUST. Big, small, there's room for them all! Celebrate your girls whether they're large and round or small and perky. Be sure to give props to your nipples; they're at the core of feminine beauty and a pleasure point, too.

TUMMY. A sexy stomach deserves loving attention, and yours is sexy whether it's a tight washboard, a kissably soft rolling bump, or a tummy adorned with a darling out-y belly button. Love yours just as it is.

BUNS. As with boobs, beautiful bums come in all shapes. Pay homage to your specially shaped buns with a frisky double hand slap. (Sound effects make this one more fun!)

LEGS. There's nothing like a great pair of gams, and they come in all sorts of shapes and sizes, too. Beyoncé-like thighs that can grip a partner are worth praising in the mirror, as are lean legs that can slide into any pair of jeans. Maybe it's your sexy calves you give love to, or even your knees. Short or tall, lean or stocky, give it up to your legs and don't hold back!

Well done, Goddess! The more you work with this sexy ritual, the more you're going to come into your fabulous, flirty self and truly own the confident, stunning creature that you are. And just like with any relationship, make sure your ritual doesn't get stale! Mix it up, invent new things to say and do, and see how much further you can take it on your own!

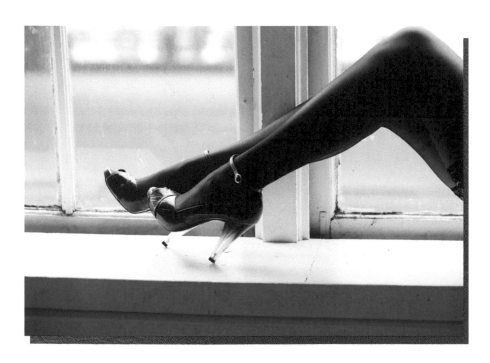

ABOUT DANA

As the Founder of Booty Parlor, Dana B. Myers has changed the lives of thousands of women by inspiring them to boost their sexy self-confidence and create sexier, more satisfying experiences, inside and outside of the bedroom.

Dana is an award-winning product developer, entrepreneur and media personality. Her advice and Booty Parlor's products have been featured in Cosmopolitan, Marie Claire, Women's Health, Self, Nylon, Parents, WWD and The Wall Street Journal. Dana has appeared on ABC Nightline, Good Morning America, Access Hollywood Live, The Wendy Williams Show and dozens of other programs.

Dana's first book, "The Official Booty Parlor Mojo Makeover: Four Weeks to a Sexier You" (HarperCollins) is a 30-day program designed to show women of all ages how to boost their confidence, sexiness and satisfaction—whether they're in a relationship or not.

Now a mother of two, Dana is releasing her next book, "The Mommy Mojo Makeover" (Viva Editions, April 2018), a guide that inspires moms to rediscover their sensuality and reignite the spark in their relationship.

Born and raised in Chicago, Dana earned a Master's Degree in Business & Entertainment from NYU and now resides in Miami with her husband/business partner, Charlie, and their two children.

Visit Dana at: www.danabmyers.com

Check out Booty Parlor at: www.bootyparlor.com ✳

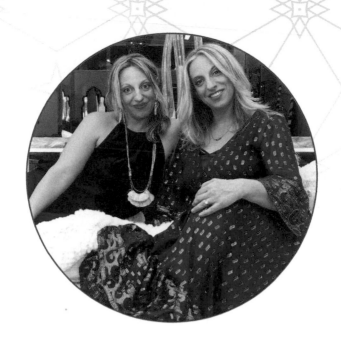

Self Love

NEW &
FULL MOON
RITUALS

✳

Divinely Contributed by

THE ASTROTWINS

Introduction

I HAVE TO BE HONEST HERE. I WAS HIGHLY
SKEPTICAL ABOUT ASTROLOGY AND
anything else that felt woo-woo until my mid 20's. Of course, I knew I
was a Libra, and somewhere in my spiritual DNA, that resonated with
me. That was as far as my depth of knowledge went when it came to
the mystery of the stars and planets. When I met other Libras, we
would hi-five each other and agreed that our parents had stellar taste
to birth us in this zodiac sign!

One snowy evening, I happened to be at my sister Tali's holiday
party and she had a copy of their book around. My then-boyfriend
persistently requested that I read about our signs' compatibility. Gasp!!
Holy Moly! Everything they said about a Libra was spot on. Loves
people, surrounds him/her self with beauty, art, and lives for being a
social butterfly—CHECK! Hates to be alone, hopeless romantic, and
can't make up their mind—YUP—that's the truth meter on 100!

I became obsessed with learning the unique make-up of each
sign. The thrill of schooling myself about the astrological quirks of
my friends and family sparked conversations that went on for hours.
I became fixated on guessing people's birth dates upon meeting
them for the very first time. Often I could pick out subtle yet obvious
characteristics that had me know for sure when I was dealing with a

Capricorn or a Gemini. Needless to say, my sisters got flooded with loaded questions about moon signs, rising signs, retrogrades, and Saturn returns!

The thing I began to appreciate most about astrology was that it gives you approval to own your SHIT! From your extraordinary qualities to the things about you that drive folks crazy. Instead of trying to change yourself into something you will never be, and going down the rabbit hole of CRAY CRAY, you begin to develop a compassionate level of self-acceptance for the ways the stars made you. On days when I feel freakin' completely off and I'm questioning everything around me, I read my horoscope that evening, only to find out that—of course—there is some damn planet in retrograde!

Astrology and the ways we are all connected to the beautiful moon cycles have a great deal to do with developing a stronger connection to our own self-love. It has much to do with the healing powers of letting go, as well as getting quiet and listening to our delicious heart-fulfilled desires. Get ready to howl at that moon, goddesses, and dive deeper into your hearts' desires with the AstroTwins, as they share their years of knowledge on how to create New Moon/Full Moon rituals! ✳

WE THINK OF THE CHART AS A BLUEPRINT OF YOUR SOUL.

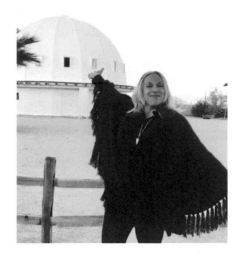

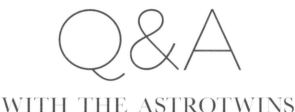

Q&A

WITH THE ASTROTWINS

L: How do you think women who are often so frustrated with their emotional states can, through understanding astrology, create a closer connection with self-love?

AT: The astrological chart is a map of where all the planets—plus the Sun and moon—were at your exact moment of birth. How it all comes together is totally unique. Fascinating fact: Only someone born at the same minute in the same time zone as you will share your chart. Even we twins, born four minutes apart, have slightly different charts. We think of the chart as a blueprint of your soul.

(MERCURY RETROGRADES) AREN'T TOTAL DISASTERS; IN FACT, RETROGRADES ARE GREAT TIMES FOR ALL THINGS 'RE' FOCUSED SUCH AS REVIEWING, REVISING, AND REUNITING.

Understanding what makes you tick from a cosmic perspective can help you live with greater awareness so you don't keep tripping over the same potholes again and again. You can also use astrology for timing and planning. It's great to look ahead and be able to prepare for challenge periods and opportunity periods—both of which are meant to help us grow.

L: **Can you share what a moon sign and rising sign are, and, say, why two Geminis with different moons and risings may appear to be the total opposite of each other?**

AT: Most people know their Sun sign, which reveals your overarching personality. The Sun sign is what you'll read in a newspaper horoscope or a magazine. But we also have a moon sign, Venus sign, Mercury sign, etc. To discover these, you have to cast a birth (natal) chart, which you can do for free on our website: astrostyle. com/free-chart. You'll need your time, date and place of birth to run an accurate natal chart.

The moon sign indicates your emotional nature which, as women, is a source of our power and strength. It can be totally different or similar to your Sun sign. In our case, we were born with the Sun in Sagittarius which makes us adventurous and entrepreneurial. But our moon sign is Scorpio, which draws us to more mystical subjects like astrology and can make us a bit more private, preferring close, intimate relationships.

The rising sign is the sign that was on the horizon line of the chart (the 9 o'clock point) at your moment of birth. You'll need to know your exact birth time to get an accurate read on this as the rising sign changes every 2-3 hours. This reveals your first responses to situations and the first impression you make on other people. The rising sign also influences your personal style and how you like to be seen in public.

L: **Why does Mercury retrograde affect our spiritual states and how can we best implement self-care during this time?**

AT: Mercury retrograde periods happen 3-4 times per year when the Earth and Mercury pass each other in their orbit. Like two trains passing at different speeds, this can create the illusion of one moving backwards. During Mercury retrograde phases, all things associated with Mercury seem to go in reverse: communication, transportation and the travel of information. These are times when squabbles start over the smallest provocation, we send a sext to our sister instead of our sweetheart (glug), traffic delays make us late to the airport—where we discover our flight has been rerouted. Mercury retrogrades last, on average, for three weeks. They aren't total disasters; in fact, retrogrades are great times for all things "re" focused such as reviewing, revising, and reuniting. Press pause when Mercury turns retrograde and go back over plans. Take time to check in with your most important relationships and smooth over any wrinkles. Many people report that they hear from old friends and exes with greater frequency during Mercury retrograde, too—hello, reconnection!

How to Create a New/Full Moon Gathering

Tired of swimming upstream? As astrologers, we've learned that living by the natural cycles and rhythms of the universe—or planning it by the planets—can really keep you in an abundant flow. Setting intentions at new and full moons has become a regular practice for us and many of our friends. New moons represent fresh starts and beginnings, while full moons mark turning points, manifestations or closure. So it's best to initiate a project or plant those seeds at a new moon, and "harvest" or make decisions at the full moon.

While it might sound woo-woo, it's not really that "out there," if you think about it. Our ancestors planted, hunted, fished and moved by the seasons and cycles of the moon. And they survived long enough to bring us into the industrial and then the digital ages. But in our tech-driven society, it's so easy to fall out of nature's rhythms. So here's how you can tune back in:

1. WHERE TO DO IT? Let the energy guide you. For the past year and a half, we've gotten together with friends to do various rituals for each new and full moon. How we end up celebrating the moon is always a spontaneous surprise! One Pisces new moon, we found ourselves in the Nevada desert, building a fire at a dry lake bed an hour or so from Vegas. In the Hamptons for the Cancer new moon, we collected shells and even found a washed-ashore crab leg! Another time, we got crafty and included Ophi's daughter Cybele, decorating God Boxes that would hold our wishes. And for the July full moon, we've hosted two of our Become Your Own Astrologer retreats in Tulum with a circle of our participants, sealing the magical energy for the week.

2. GATHER THE TRIBE. Rally your soul-seeking and self-aware friends—and invite that person who might not be as far along on their spiritual exploration, too. (Out in the Nevada desert for one ritual, the driver who chartered us spontaneously joined our fireside circle and made the most heart-melting wish, bringing tears to everyone's eyes.) Remember, this is not an exclusionary thing, so share the love! It's great to take turns hosting if you have a regular moon crew, or to come together and each add something to the plans.

3. HAVE SUPPLIES.
   - Matches or candles to burn something you're letting go of
   - Crystals, rocks, shells or other natural artifacts—you might even want to tuck your wishes under/into one of these
   - Sage wands (also called smudge sticks), oils or Palo Santo wood to burn and "clear" the energy before you do your ritual. This can have the effect of creating a truly sacred space for setting intentions
   - Divination decks like Tarot, goddess cards or angel cards
   - A beautiful cloth for setting up a group altar
   - Photos of loved ones or cherished objects that can sit on the altar with your wishes for a "moon bath"

4. CREATE THE ATMOSPHERE. Again, you can let the spirit of the moon move you, but we've found it works to play soft music, serve invigorating food, light candles or a fire, and to create an ambience that helps people tune in and be more present. You might sit on floor cushions or go around in a circle and each say aloud what you'd like to release or manifest (at the full moon), or begin anew (at the new moon). When weather permits, an outdoor ceremony is great so you can feel tuned into nature—and hopefully even see the full moon! After everyone has made wishes or written down intentions, it's great to "break" any heaviness with music or movement. Invite the energy to lead. A new moon circle could inspire a walk, angel card readings or a fun outing to hunt for new outfits, crystals, or supplies that are needed to spur your wishes along. Your full moon gathering may turn into a dance party, a drum circle, a spontaneous swim or who knows what!

5. PUT YOUR WISHES SOMEPLACE SACRED. Some people say you should sleep with your moon wishes under your pillow. We've done it! We like to put them somewhere special, like an altar. Tali is especially into creating altars with pretty crystals and found objects—her own brand of spiritual home décor. We're inspired by beautiful store windows and displays all the time—hello, Anthropologie and Bergdorf Goodman!

How to Set Intentions or Make Moon Wishes

1. WRITE 'EM DOWN. It's not required, but putting intentions into writing can take them much further. One study even showed that people who wrote down their goals, shared them with others, and maintained accountability for their goals were 33% more likely to achieve them, versus those who just formulated goals. Which brings us to . . .

2. SHARE SOME OF YOUR WISHES WITH YOUR CIRCLE. Let's face it, our memories can lapse. Having other people hold the space (or hold you accountable) for the intentions you set at each moon can add extra power. If sharing is too personal, you can get a deck of angel cards and have each person draw one, then perhaps share a little something about what the message inspires.

3. THINK IN TWO-WEEK AND SIX-MONTH CYCLES. There is one new moon each month, followed by a full moon two weeks later. While they aren't in similar zodiac signs, the energy from the new moon actually builds up over that two-week period. The cycle basically goes like this:

SET THE INTENTION & GET TO WORK AT THE NEW MOON. The new moon gives way to that first sliver of light as the shadow moves and the moon reveals herself—or "waxes," as it's called.

REAP RESULTS OR MAKE DECISIONS AT THE FULL MOON.
Two weeks later, we have the complete illumination of the full moon, which can reveal what was in the dark. This is a time to take decisive action or to tie up loose ends and complete a project.

Finish what you started for two weeks after the full moon. After the full moon, la luna "wanes" or recedes into shadows for two weeks, a good time to deal with what came up at the full moon, wrap up loose ends, and prepare to start something new at the next new moon.

Each new moon also has a six-month astrological cycle—for example, the March new moon in Pisces always links to the September full moon in Pisces. The December/January Capricorn new moon comes full circle with a late June/July Capricorn full moon. So you can set specific intentions at a new moon, based on the energies of that zodiac sign, and watch them unfold in the coming half-year.

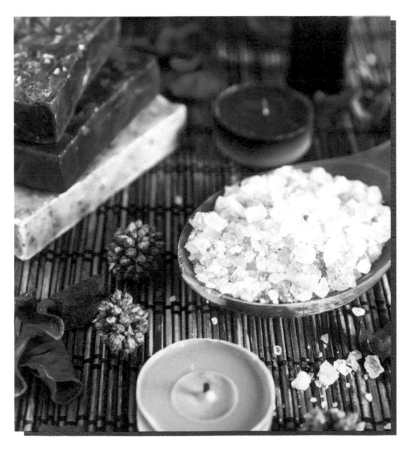

ABOUT THE ASTROTWINS

Dubbed the "astrologers to the stars," identical twin sisters Ophira and Tali Edut, known as the AstroTwins, are professional astrologers who reach millions worldwide through their spot-on predictions.

Through their website, Astrostyle.com, Ophira and Tali help "bring the stars down to earth" with their unique, lifestyle-based approach to astrology. They are also the official astrologers for Refinery29, ELLE. com, Elle Magazine (U.S.), and have read charts for celebrities including Beyoncé, Stevie Wonder, Jessica Simpson and Sting. They are regular guests on SiriusXM and have appeared on Bravo's The Real Housewives of New Jersey, doing on-air readings for the cast.

They have authored four print books: AstroStyle, Love Zodiac, Shoestrology and Momstrology (their #1 Amazon best-selling astrological parenting guide) and a growing collection of eBooks, including their popular annual horoscope guides.

Visit the AstroTwins at: www.astrostyle.com ✳

"

OUT IN THE NEVADA
DESERT FOR ONE
RITUAL, THE DRIVER
WHO CHARTERED
US SPONTANEOUSLY
JOINED OUR FIRESIDE
CIRCLE AND MADE
THE MOST HEART-
MELTING WISH,
BRINGING TEARS
TO EVERYONE'S EYES.

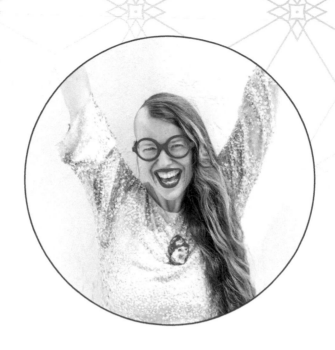

Self Love

#SOULSPARKLE:
THE JOURNEY TO CLAIM OUR WORTH IN THE WORLD & SHINE BRIGHT

✳

Divinely Contributed by

LAINIE LOVE DALBY

Introduction

LAINIE IS ONE OF THOSE WOMEN WHO
CATCHES YOUR EYE WITH HER BOLD SELF—
expression. She gives permission to all of us who long to wear two-toned, bright neon leggings, a one shoulder sequin top, and rock the shit out of a feathery boa. You long to pull her close to you and ask her what her secret is—*How do you live out loud with zero fucks given?!*

As I've gotten to know the many layers of Lainie Love, I have come to find out she is part wizard, part goddess and all holy healer.

Her deep reverence for the underdog is so needed in a world that often only wants to see the "perfect," shiny, beautiful parts of us while it shuns anything that is "freakish, dark, or abnormal" by society's standards. Lainie Love has the ability to focus her multi-colored, glitter-encrusted wand on peeling back old, unneeded layers of self-judgment and shame. Her stand for all of us women is to live in our full TRUTH and step just as audaciously into our purpose.

Adjust your crowns and place a hand on your heart, as we explore a fun and empowered way to RISE into our full and unique #SOULSPARKLE, as she likes to call it. Raise your other fist into the air as we call in our ancestors to help reclaim our self-worth and stand in our power through Lainie Love's potent ritual! ✳

"

TOGETHER,
I BELIEVE WE CAN
BUILD A KINDER,
BRAVER & MORE
BEAUTIFUL
WORLD—BUT
WITHOUT LOVING
OURSELVES &
CLAIMING OUR
WORTH FIRST, WE
CAN'T EVEN BEGIN
THE JOURNEY.

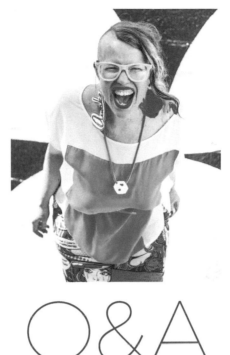

Q&A

WITH LAINIE LOVE DALBY

L: Your own journey, Lainie, is such a picture of what it feels like to embody the path of self-love. A lot of times, we feel the pressure to show only the fluffy, feel-good side of our lives, and bypass the dark side of the RLS (REAL LIFE SHIT!) that is happening. Can you lead us through some moments that you danced with your darkness that galvanized you to do the work you are now doing?

LD: Growing up as an obese and wildly creative child led me to a vicious cycle of yo-yo dieting and gaining and losing over 1,300 pounds in my lifetime. This caused me to feel uncomfortable in my own skin and body, never feeling worthy or good enough as I was. I was also bullied almost every year in school and never felt like I fit in anywhere. After years of emotional and psychological abuse, I internalized this language of violence, eventually turning the abuse against myself in the form of self-hatred. I had forgotten who I was—a Divine child of the Great Goddess—and why I was here at this most crucial time in human history. I had gotten wholly distracted from what matters most.

This lasted until a near brush with death's door catalyzed my spiritual journey almost a decade ago, landing me in an intensive Interfaith Seminary program at One Spirit in NYC. Yet it took my recent "Divine reality check" with illness during 2015 and 2016 to truly shift my perspective and daily actions.

IN THE END, I LIKE TO REMEMBER THAT THE BODY IS JUST AN ELABORATE CLOAK FOR THE SOUL.

I know intimately now that my body is a sacred vessel, an exquisite temple, a holy sanctuary, and that I am a unique imprint of the Divine. There will never be another me, with my innate #SOULSPARKLE. My illness catalyzed a total reframe, a conscious choice to break the oppressive and limiting patriarchal chains and ditch dieting for good. In its place, I fully embody a radical lifestyle shift each day that involves deeply nourishing my body, heart and soul, giving her what she needs to THRIVE. I came back home to my body and to the earth, connecting back to my innate wildness and what it means to be deeply in touch with my core essence and fierce feminine fire within. Now, I help other women to do the same.

In the end, I like to remember that *the body is just an elaborate cloak for the soul.* And the soul is yearning to be brought into its fullest expression in this lifetime. It desires to reach its peak (r) evolutionary potential for the good of all in our global village. Like the oak tree encoded in the acorn, the map to our destiny and deepest truths lies deep within our bodies.

This is crucial to understand because each of us MATTERS, and we're here to DO something that matters. We're all artists here to co-create our lives as a great masterpiece for the good of all! Together, I believe we can build a kinder, braver and more beautiful world—but without loving ourselves and claiming our worth FIRST, we can't even begin the journey.

This is why I've made it my mission to free human spirits that have been oppressed and devalued to Sparkle Shamelessly® and step into their power through guided ceremonial journeys and safe spaces of sisterhood that catalyze deep healing, growth and transformation. We come together to remember who we are and step into our (r)evolutionary potential TOGETHER in Beloved Community. Essentlally, I hold space for others to RISE.

L: **As an entry point for someone who is just beginning their self-love research, where do you recommend they begin?**

LD: The way I made it through was by being extremely GENTLE wlth myself. I was clear that none of my actions were going to be "quick fixes," as the media likes to falsely promise us. I knew I was embarking on a lifelong journey, starting one step at a time, with one foot in front of the other. I found that a daily practice of deep and radical hospitality towards myself and my body helped to carry me through.

I also began to research the root cause of my long history with self-hatred and separation from my core essence. I wanted to know WHY I had become severed from myself. This led me straight down the path of reclaiming the ancient Goddess tradition and the Divine Feminine that was stamped out by the patriarchy. We women have been silenced, shamed, burned, and continuously kept bound for centuries. Even the epidemic of violence against women and girls today is a symptom of this collective amnesia.

I needed to literally wake up and return to my roots as a woman, reclaiming my Priestess lineage and innate power. I began learning about the spiritual path of my ancestors and cultivating the wild feminine within myself. I also needed a deep restoration and rebalancing of the masculine and feminine energies within myself, since our society is so heavily imbalanced towards the linear, product-driven masculine.

OUR TASK ALONG THE JOURNEY IS TO REMEMBER THAT SOMEONE OUT THERE NEEDS US. THE QUESTION IS, ARE WE GOING TO LIVE OUR LIVES SO THEY CAN FIND US?

In my own personal state of imbalance, I had learned to become a bulldozer (a condition familiar to those of us who live in NYC), bringing my masculine energy to the forefront and just pushing through: through the suffering, through the excess pounds, through the joint and knee pains, through my gastrointestinal distress, through my deep lack of self-worth. In order to heal, I had to bring the sacred feminine back into balance within myself and truly learn the Sacred Arts of surrender, slowing down, tapping into my deep well of intuition and being in the flow with all of life.

Each moment I began to welcome the journey and made the fundamental daily shifts of treating my body as a sacred temple, practicing forgiveness and radical acceptance of what is, moving towards deep nourishment, engaging in deep ritual and ceremony, and most of all *remembering to Sparkle Shamelessly®*.

Sparkling Shamelessly is one of my signature Sacred Arts that I teach. At its most basic, it's allowing our spiritual magnificence to come forth—our authentic soul essence, and the reality and raw truth of who we are in each moment. It's being authentic, UNAPOLOGETIC, and fiercely aligned. It's a great *remembering*, calling all the parts of ourselves back in. It's an innate *knowing* that we are walking stardust and that our true nature is to shine bright, together creating a constellation that lights up the world.

THE INNER CRITIC WILL INEVITABLY RETURN, SOMETIMES BRINGING THE DARKNESS WITH IT IN TOW. I CALL MINE J.E.F.F.R.Y.

L: **Once we begin to live in a world where we are learning to love ourselves and claim our worth, I find that we are often met with resistance. There are days we don't want to get out of bed and be kind to ourselves. What practices or wisdom can you share that can support us through those moments?**

LD: The inner critic will inevitably return, sometimes bringing the darkness with it in tow. I call mine **J.E.F.F.R.Y**. He symbolizes **J**udgment, **E**go, **F**ear, **F**ailure, **R**esistance and **Y**ielding. I notice him with compassion and observe his irrational behavior, and then I bring in the voice of **W.I.L.M.A.** to the rescue. She's **W**isdom, **I**ntuition, **L**aughter, **M**astery, and **A**uthenticity. She just laughs off his ridiculous banter, and helps me to center back into the truth of who I really am: a badass sorcerer of Divine light who's Motherf*@!ing POWERFUL!

There are also the outer critics who may come for us when we start living our full truth and standing in our authentic power. They may come at us with "BITCH," or insert-any-other-derogatory-name-here.

In some cases it's really just society's modern day version of labeling a powerful woman as a WITCH and finding a way to persecute her. I like to do a reframe and think of **B.I.T.C.H.** as an acronym: **B**adass **I**n **T**otal **C**ontrol of **H**erself.

With all that said, we must claim our worth in the world, because if we don't, no one else will. What I mean by that is not allowing the outside world to define us, repress us, hold us back or tell us what we can and cannot do. Instead, we need to see our true beauty and gifts from the inside out and claim our worth from this place of deep soul knowing. We must learn to source a deep inner sense of value instead of seeking outer validation. The invitation is to dance with the resistance and remind ourselves of our inherent brilliance and gifts even in the most difficult moments.

Our task along the journey is to remember that someone out there needs us. The question is, *Are we going to live our lives so they can find us?*

When you truly believe that you're worthy and own the unique #SOULSPARKLE deep within yourself, then the negative banter just becomes ridiculous. You have to remember with fierce conviction that your playing small doesn't serve anyone, least of all yourself. We each have a Divine Legacy that only we can bring. The moment-by-moment invitation is to refocus on what matters most: living into our full (r)evolutionary potential for the good of everyone in our global village.

Ready to join me in Sparkling SHAMELESSLY, sister?!

A Ritual of Remembrance for Claiming Self-Worth

I begin by consciously creating a sacred space through intention. Then I plant my feet firmly on the ground in a power stance, my legs a bit wider than my shoulders. I place one hand on my abdomen and one hand on my heart, then take a few deep 4-count breaths to help get out of my head (and my own way) and, instead, root back into my body and heart. I actually visualize roots growing out through the soles of my feet and base of my spine (or root chakra), connecting into our Great Mother Earth beneath me. I send these roots all the way down into her molten fiery core to ground me fully and then slowly draw this energy and fire up into my belly (or solar plexus chakra).

I then close my eyes and call in my angels, ancestors, guides and any other benevolent forces to hold me and help me to remember who I am. As Mama Oprah has said, *"I embody the line from Maya Angelou's poem 'Our Grandmothers,' where she says, 'I come as one, but I stand as 10,000.'"* We stand on the shoulders of giants who risked everything for us to be here today. I live with them, breathe with them and call on them often for guidance as I remember that our ancestors deeply desire for us to self-actualize in this lifetime for the good of all. We have the opportunity to consciously carry on the legacy of our lineage. I continuously choose to anchor this deep wisdom into my body.

After this prayer, I say a mantra to raise my vibration: *"You're here because you're supposed to be. You MATTER. You are worthy. Know that someone out there needs you. You must live your life so they can find you. Go forth & SPARKLE SHAMELESSLY®!"*

I continue with *"I am"* on each in-breath, and *"F*@!ing powerful"* on each out-breath, over and over until I truly feel it deep in every cell of my body. You can insert the words *"I am . . . limitless"* or any other rendition that suits you and makes your soul sing. To close the ritual, I place my hands in prayer pose and offer a deep bow of gratitude and then I bend down and place my hands on Mother Earth to thank her for her constant support and sustenance. And voila! You have an instant inner pep talk that you can use anytime, anywhere (even in a bathroom stall before a big meeting)!

The truth is that, when we fundamentally love and accept ourselves for who we are, no matter what that looks like, we can push past all the BS (**B**elief **S**ystems) in society and get to the business of truly living fully and Sparkling SHAMELESSLY. We are a miraculous creation: Our bodies work tirelessly on our behalf. Just think that our hearts beat over 100,000 times in ONE DAY for us alone. We are so blessed to have this one wild and precious life. Who are we NOT to love, honor and revere this vessel that allows us to be alive on earth, here and now?

To help you continue the journey of claiming your worth in the world, I have a parting gift for you: the #SOULSPARKLE Starter Kit. It's a 13-day free course designed as an interactive journey to radical self-acceptance and the courage to just be UNAPOLOGETICALLY YOU in the world.

Get access at www.LainieLoveDalby.com!

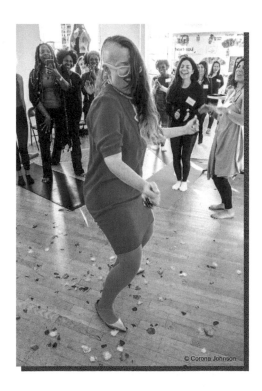

© Corona Johnson

ABOUT LAINIE

Lainie Love Dalby is a Sacred Artist, Embodied Leadership Mentor & (R)evolutionary Muse on a mission to free human spirits that have been oppressed and devalued to Sparkle SHAMELESSLY® & step into their power. As a spiritual thought leader with her own brand of multimedia ministry, she is dismantling old systems, ideas and ways of being that promote separateness and limit our full (r)evolutionary potential.

She is also deeply passionate about ending the violence we perpetrate against each other and our own bodies by reminding us of our inherent Divinity within and helping to bring the sacred Feminine back into balance in our own lives and the world. Like a modern day medicine woman, her ultimate goal is to help us feel more comfortable in our own skin and live in greater alignment with who we truly are by unleashing our bold creativity, innate wildness & fierce feminine courage.

*She is the founder of **#SOULSPARKLE,** a holistic lifestyle and spiritual development company helping women & the LGBTQ community become leaders of change and co-create their lives as a great masterpiece for the good of all. They create sacred arts education and immersion experiences to catalyze personal healing & transformation so we can build a kinder, braver & more beautiful world together. As global ritualist Barbara Biziou has said, "Like a great sculpture, Lainie Love can see what lives inside of you and frees it to live fully."*

Visit Lainie Love at: www.LainieLoveDalby.com ✳

2

LUSCIOUS MOVEMENT

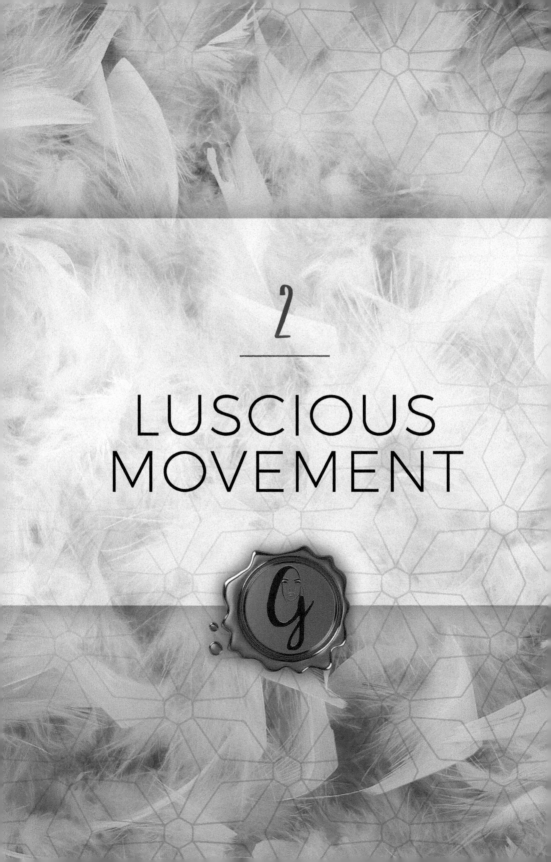

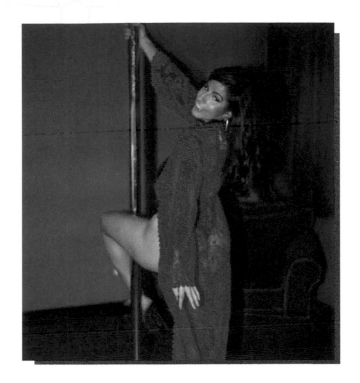

I WAS BAMBOOZLED! Why had glossy pages of magazines brainwashed so many of us women into thinking that going to the gym and working ourselves into a hot, sweaty mess would be the cure for our distress? Never teaching us to get out of our heads in this linear way of thinking and, instead, feel into our bodies, where all the answers are held. We are not taught to move this wise vessel in a way that feels like heaven for us. *Did you know that some slow, lingering hip circles, along with an irrestistible playlist can send you into a state of ecstasy?*

It is time to reclaim that connection to our bodies that has been lost!

For years I thought my goal for going to the gym would be this teeny-tiny body-which isn't possible with my gorgeous ass curves.

I went to the gym faithfully and found myself flipping from page to page of the magazines with body envy. Even worse, I was carrying around loads of body *shame*. What I truly needed was some wise priestess to gently guide me and say, "Your body is gorgeous! The way your back arches is a spectacular piece of art! Learn to love every part with gentle ease. Start by indulging in lots of rest, slowing down on the wine and champagne, and tune in to what your body is truly calling for."

I had believed the masculine route was the way to my body's health. At age 18, I signed up for my first gym membership at good ol' Fitness USA. Detroit's all-women gym, where most of the members came just for the complimentary Jacuzzi and steam room (that seemed to always be out of order). Goddess bless those "trainers" who totally sold me the dream that, if I did 30 minutes of daily cardio, I was guaranteed to have a Beyoncé body. I'm sure they were just giving the sales pitch that some patriarchal boss told them to—the goal was to sell as many memberships in a day as possible, right?—not realizing the damage that can be done to women who already live in a body-obsessed society.

I BELIEVE WHEN A WOMAN HAS ACCESS TO HER BODY, SHE HAS ACCESS TO HER TRUTH.

That Beyhive body? Well, that never happened! As time went on I became more and more resigned from believing that I would ever have a body I adored; one that I could look in the mirror and wink at. I started binge eating to numb the emotional pain. This inevitably lead to my fabulous inner critic *who loved* to obsess about my food trauma for hours on end. I began to dislike myself a little bit more each day. When I went out to celebratory dinners with girlfriends, my joy would quickly turn sour! I found myself analyzing and stressing over each ingredient on the menu, and then would beat myself up if I didn't choose the "healthiest option"! After 14 years of pushing myself to search for something that wasn't meant to be, an idea was planted. Maybe this was the body I was supposed to live in and love! Could there be another way to find acceptance for myself?

Divine intervention at its finest happened a few days later. Rochelle Schieck, the founder of Qoya, was sharing office space with my sister. Lucky me! One day she began to speak about this new way to experience *movement*, and I could feel my whole body tingle. Was this one of those messages you get at the exact moment you're ready to receive it? I shared my desire to attend, she gave me the details—and I was there!

That first Qoya experience reconnected me to the divine feminine energy inside that was dying to come out and play! Qoya became my weekly movement ritual, which led me to Bernadette Pleasant, the founder of Femme!™. Suddenly, I was attracting classes at lightening speed that were all about ME feeling delicious in my body!

But my own body was often SO anxious that I couldn't luxuriate fully in these moments. I was doing all of this sensual movement, and sometimes I couldn't turn my brain off—or the fear that was running through my body. Working with The Lara Touch helped me to clear these emotions out so I could deepen my relationship with trust and pleasure.

The process became even more enticing as I began to worship each mouth-watering curve, which magnetized lovers and romantic partners who did the same. Learning to accept my full range of feelIngs was Incredibly healing. Moving my body in these slow, savory, circular motions would invite golden tears to come up and gently splash my face.

One of my favorites is the fierce cat cow roll at S Factor. It feels like a huge release—as you let go of whatever is feeling stuck inside at that moment. And Bernadette's oh so powerful sacred ritual for honoring grief and rage? There is nothing like it!

MOVING MY BODY IN WAYS THAT FEEL LIKE HOME HAS BEEN ONE OF THE SIMPLEST YET MOST ELUSIVE GIFTS. It's my connection to sheer JOY! I believe that, when a woman has access to her body, she has access to her truth.

Discovering how to give myself my own loving touch has stopped me from seeking out lovers who could sense my big, lustful appetite. It saved me from wanting to pull all my hair out when I had a small, crying baby.

My body is now my compass.

I feel this "buried treasure"—our bodies—is something that we as women need to reclaim. We have to learn what feels like paradise to us first, before we can guide anyone else to touch the temple of a goddess. We need to explore why we *stopped* moving our bodies in this way. And most importantly, we need to grant ourselves permission to slow down and relish the time we spend moving in a relaxed state.

Goddesses! One of my deepest desires is for you to explore your dreamland, which is full of pure pleasure just for you! I have four of the most genius body whisperers to lead you gently back into the place we often vacate. Close your eyes, lick your lips ever so slowly, and relish each leisure second as you begin to get acquainted with BLISS! ✳

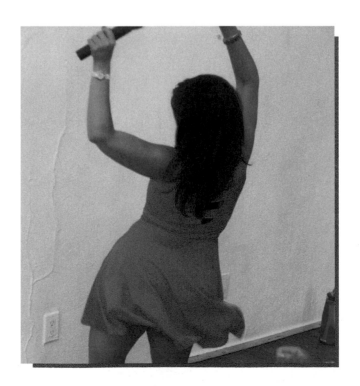

"

MOVING MY
BODY IN WAYS
THAT FEEL LIKE
HOME HAS
BEEN ONE OF
THE SIMPLEST
YET MOST
ELUSIVE GIFTS.

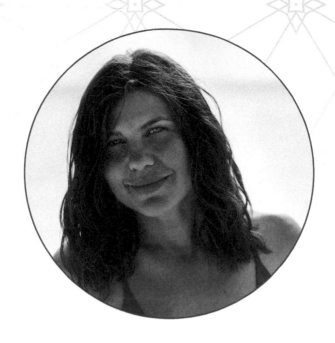

Luscious Movement

A SHIFT IN
CONSCIOUSNESS

Divinely Contributed by

ROCHELLE SCHIECK

Introduction

QOYA WAS THE BEGINNING OF ME CREATING
A CONNECTION WITH MY BODY. I TRUSTED
Rochelle, so her invitation to come experience the class was met
with little resistance. I felt some sort of energy flirting with my body,
tempting my senses and enticing my interest. It was as if something
was calling my name!

I can remember my first experience with Qoya at the Bhakti
Center. I ran from 2nd to 1st Avenue on a busy NYC morning, my heart
pounding with nervous excitement—paired with the fear of running
late. I had invited a high strung Virgo friend to meet me there, and I
didn't want to disappoint myself or her by missing the beginning of our
first class.

Finally, arriving out of breath—my eyes scanned the stairs leading
up to the studio. Luscious, full, red rose petals were carefully placed
on each stair leading all the way up to the door. I can still feel my
body's reaction—I felt at home, enlivened. I was curious about what
else might be revealed during this experience.

Deep in my well of pleasure, I got an intuitive hit, that this wasn't
going to be your "average dance class"!

Rochelle helped us from the very moment we began to move out
of our heads and drop into the sheer delight of our bodies. Her words

melted into my skin: "Whatever feels good, do that. If I say move your left hand and your right hand wants to move, honor that."

A rush of approval washed over my entire body. Damn, that felt fucking amazing! She broke down some body wisdom that felt like a lover whispering in my ear: "We are three parts wise, wild, and free." For a person who felt lost inside of her body most days, this adventure was like meeting the forgotten wisdoms of the goddess.

Savoring that day gave me evidence that there was so much more to be found within the truth of our bodies. Rochelle is an alchemist when it comes to evoking trapped emotions in our bodies. Breathe with me, my goddess sisters, as she invites you on the journey inside of *you*. ✷

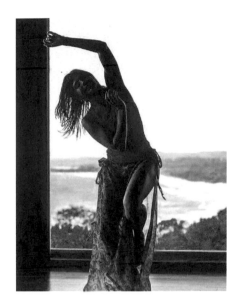

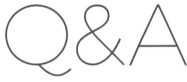

WITH ROCHELLE SCHIECK

L: **What stirs up your rapture when it comes to women?**

R: Their resilience. Women are such deep feeling creatures. In the midst of life's blessings and challenges, I'm touched by women who keep expanding their heart and choosing love again and again. There are so many invitations to close down, give up or become cynical, but I find most of the women I encounter use their struggles and sadness as fuel for compassion and empathy. Love is powerful medicine and I am a believer in the power of it.

L: Why do you think movement is such a healing force and shakes up the entire way we have previously viewed our lives?

R: The body doesn't lie. The way our mind works is by judging the past or anticipating the future. The way our body processes information is in the present moment. Movement is healing, because all healing takes place by simply coming into the present moment.

L: What is your secret wish for all women in the world?

R: My wish for all women in the world is to feel the physical sensation of truth in their body and to have the freedom to follow that, express that, and live that in the world. To trust themselves and enjoy their journey, remembering that our essence as women, as goddesses, is wise, wild and free.

This is the main idea in Qoya—that, through movement, we remember our essence is wise, wild and free. *Wise, wild and free* also draws reference to the movement forms that we practice in Qoya.

Wise draws on the wisdom of yoga. Wild, the creative expression in dance. And *free*—expanding our capacity to enjoy being in our body through sensual movement. Through this practice, we learn how to use movement as a portal to remembering our deepest truths and the physical sensation of being aligned with that truth. Then we learn *how to set that feeling as north on our compasses.*

_____

Becoming Wise, Wild and Free
Day 1 from 10 Days to Love Qoya

MOVE

Let's do an experiment to see if this is true for you:

For the next 30 seconds, shake your right hand intensely.
As fast as you can.
- Get wild with it.
- Really shake. *(Shake it like a Polaroid picture . . .)*
- Remember to breathe—take two more deep breaths as you shake your right hand only.
- Now stop.

Gently cup both hands in front of your chest as if you were holding a ball.
- Feel the difference between your right hand and your left hand.
- Feel how one hand is stronger and at the same time lighter.
- Feel how one is more dull and less animated.
- How do your right and left hands feel different?

Next, we'll apply that same idea to activate each part of your body and feel your whole body more awake, alive and energized.
- Make it simple.
- Just turn on your current favorite song and shake each part of your body, moving through your whole body, for 3-5 minutes.

Shake for about 10-15 seconds your:
- feet
- legs
- hips
- torso
- shoulders
- arms
- whole body

Or—shake along with me in the video!

AND NOW, MY GIFT TO YOU:

Go online to: http://www.qoya.love/10-days-intro/ and access all ten days of movement!

If you fall in love with Qoya—and yourself all over again, as I know you will—you can then check out a class near you and celebrate with other goddesses!

There are over 150 certified Qoya teachers and classes, workshops and retreats scheduled worldwide. We invite all of you goddesses to join us—either virtually or in full physical embodiment!

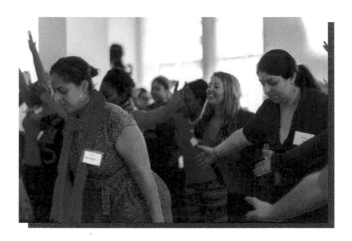

ABOUT ROCHELLE

Rochelle Schieck is the founder of Qoya. Qoya combines movement, ritual, community and pilgrimage for women. Since its inception in 2009, she has trained hundreds of Qoya teachers, taught thousands of Qoya movement classes, and led dozens of retreats in the most sacred places on earth with one intention in mind: to remember, and to help others do the same. Her work has been featured in outlets like New York Magazine, Oprah.com, The Telegraph, and Psychology Today. To learn more you can visit: www.qoya.love and read her book titled Qoya: A Compass for Navigating an Embodied Life that is Wise, Wild and Free.

Visit Rochelle at: www.qoya.love ✳

"

OUR ESSENCE
AS WOMEN,
AS GODDESSES,
IS WISE, WILD
AND FREE.

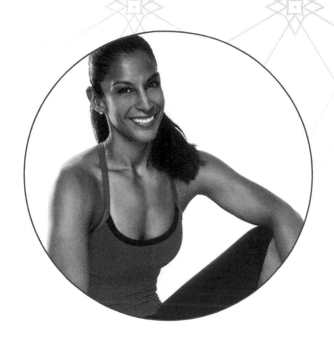

Luscious Movement

A WHOLE
NEW LEVEL

Divinely Contributed by

PATRICIA MORENO

Introduction

AS WOMEN, WE HAVE COME TO A TIME WHERE WE ARE SO OVER THE HARD-CORE, masculine, competing workouts! We are ready to say buh-bye to being so sore from working our goddess bods that we can't even get out of bed the next morning! Our desire is to feel an ultimate connection to our bodies through feminine and spiritual movements. We want to leave the room feeling inspired and deliciously good about ourselves after a workout.

The first time I took Patricia's self-created intenSati, my whole body tingled with delight. Every inch of my body felt energized! I loved the high-fiving and how she had us all cheering each other on. By the time it was over, something had been stirred inside of me—inside all of us!

One of my yummiest experiences with Patricia was at our April 21, 2013 Goddess On The Go event. She had us form two lines facing each other. At that moment, we were able to truly see the other person: Their happiness, their self-doubts, any grief that they may have been feeling. We created an intention to bring to ourselves and the goddess we were with on this journey. We shared our loving words for one another back and forth: "You are awesome!" "You are powerful!" "You are loved." By the time class was over, there was not a dry eye in the room.

"

IT IS SUCH A PRIVILEGE TO BE HUMAN.

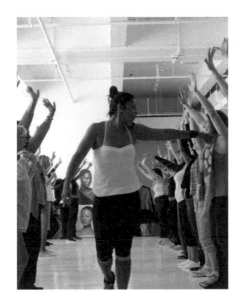

Q&A

WITH PATRICIA MORENO

L: **How can we change the outdated mindset of women who think they have to spend hours struggling at the gym?**

P: If we want to change how we feel about ourselves, we need practices and rituals. For so many, exercise is something we do to fix or punish ourselves. When we exercise because we love our body or our selves, and we start with a positive reason why, it makes something we have to do become something we love to do.

IT'S MY JOB TO STAY INSPIRED AND EVOLVING.

L: Why is doing a movement we love so important and how does that align with other parts of our lives?

P: It is such a privilege to be human. When we do things daily that help us connect to the full spectrum of who we are, I believe it leads to a better life. intenSati is intended to be a way for people to change the reason why they exercise. Instead of exercising to achieve "thinner thighs in 30 days," exercising becomes a means by which to achieve a life you love in a body you love. If you want to live a life you love in a body you love, it begins with loving the one you have, and we practice doing that while working out hard, meditating, performing incantations, aerobics and intention setting.

L: What inspires you to continuously be this creative, genius force?

P: I love to learn and I love to teach. I keep myself inspired by learning more about ways to help people create lasting positive change in their lives—and I practice on myself. It's my job to stay inspired and evolving.

A Ritual to Wake Up and RISE!

WAKE UP AND RISE! This is a 7 to 10-minute morning routine that will help you raise your vibration and impregnate your subconscious mind with positive vibes that will lead to positive changes in your body and your life.

Songs: "Rise" by Katy Perry, "Rise" by Selena Gomez & "Rise" by Danny Gokey

STEP ONE: "Rise" by Katy Perry

Begin by sitting in a chair or on the floor and focusing on your heart center. Breathe slowly in and out. Put your intention on moving into a state of non-judgmental awareness and unconditional love. Imagine all blocks are removed from your path.

Mentally affirm: "Every day in a very true way, I co-create my reality. As above, so is below, this is what I know."

   Mentally see yourself without limitations and already who you want to be. Rise up to your next level of health and well-being.

1 minute: Start with a 1-minute square breath. Breathe in for four counts. Hold your breath for four counts. Exhale four counts. Hold the breath out for four counts. This will help you bring good vibes to your body and mind.

2 minutes: March with exaggerated arm swings, bringing your knees as high as possible. Inhale three segmented breaths or sniffs in through the nose and exhale on the fourth count through the mouth with a HA! As you march, stay on the balls of your feet to stimulate the pressure points on the ball of the foot, heart, lung and thyroid gland.

2 minutes: Power lunge and push kick YES I CAN! Lunge to the right side, bring your feet together, kick your right foot like you are pushing open a door. Every time you kick say, "YES I CAN!"
Repeat for 1 minute on the left side.

STEP TWO: "Rise" by Selena Gomez (1 minute song)

Minute 6: Start in a chair pose. Say, "I am ready to rise," then crawl out to a plank pose.

Hold and say, "I am ready to rise."

Do two pushups on your knees or toes and say, "I am ready to rise."

Crawl back to a standing forward bend and say, "I am ready to rise."

Repeat for 1 minute.

STEP THREE: "Rise" by Danny Gokey (1 minute song) Cobra to baby pose: Do a cobra pose—shining your heart forward, and imagine the sun filling up your heart with light.

Smile and mentally affirm: "I am grateful for this day."

Inhale and exhale three times.

Slowly move back into baby pose. Place your forehead on the floor as you stimulate the frontal lobe, the good decision-making part of your brain, and mentally affirm:

"Thank you for my life. I am glad I am alive."

Repeat three times.

STEP FOUR: Savasana

Take some time to lie on your back and imagine every cell of your body filled with unconditional love. Visualize yourself in perfect health and in a fit and strong body.

Rehearse your day mentally and see yourself succeeding and making loving and positive choices for yourself.

Walk forward confidently in the direction of your dreams and you will find everything is aligned, and that synchronicities are happening all the time. You are blessed.

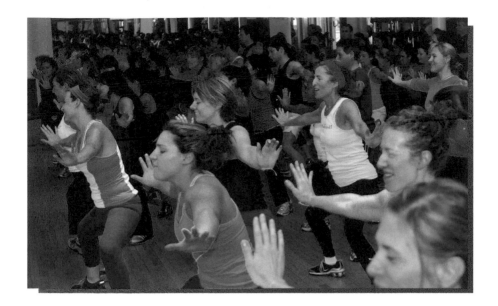

ABOUT PATRICIA

Patricia Moreno has been training, mentoring and educating people all over the world for over 30 years. In an effort to end her own struggle with weight, eating disorders and body image issues, she created The intenSati Method, a life transforming workout which combines her expertise in fitness, dance, martial arts, yoga, nutrition, meditation and spiritual practices.

Encouraged by her own transformation, and the life changing stories of her students, Patricia has gone on to create several other workouts, courses, and workshops including yogaSati, warriorSati, coreSati, danceSati and the intenSati Leadership Training. She is committed to being a powerful force for positive change in the world, and continues to find revolutionary ways to uplift her students and help them to change, inside and out. Patricia believes that through conscious, intentional living, a commitment to excellence and the power of love, every person is able to live a life filled with peace, happiness and joy.

Visit Patricia at: www.satilife.com ✳

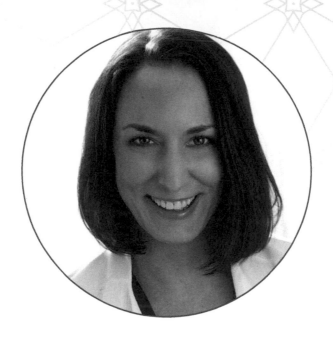

Luscious Movement

THE ULTIMATE
CHILLAX

Divinely Contributed by

LARA ANN RIGGIO

Introduction

MORE THAN ANYTHING, MOST GODDESSES
I KNOW WANT TO ACTIVATE THEIR SUPER
powers to manifest their wildest dreams. Before I joined Lara's
Believe Boot Camp, my confidence around having what I wanted was
pretty low.

The feeling and vision were in place; however, this would set my
nervous system into a panic. My underlying belief was that my life
would never get as big as I desired!

Lara used her guidess skills to clear away the anxiety and doubt
that had me paralyzed by my fears. Those late night dreams that had
been on auto replay finally began to come alive! Lara's words echo in
my mind whenever I find myself procrastinating on doing something
that scares the shit out of me: "Focus on what you want, and not on
what you don't want." As simple as that sounds, her techniques retrain
your belief/nervous system so you can make your wildest dreams and
most-sought desires into a reality. ✳

"

THE LAW OF
ATTRACTION IS A
REAL LAW OF THE
UNIVERSE. WHAT
YOU BELIEVE, YOU
CAN MANIFEST.
HOWEVER, THE LAW
OF ATTRACTION
WORKS WITH
FEELINGS,
NOT WORDS.

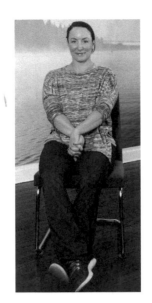

Q&A

WITH LARA RIGGIO

L: Why do you think so many people feel helpless when it comes to manifesting the desires they are most hungry for?

LR: The Law of Attraction is a real law of the Universe. What you believe, you can manifest. However, the Law of Attraction works with feelings, not words. If you are saying you believe you can make more money, but are feeling anxious while saying it, you are actually manifesting anxiety around having more money, not more money.

If your parents struggled with money, it's probable that you picked up their financial beliefs and habits; thinking you can have an abundance of money could threaten your alliance with them subconsciously. If you saw your mom unhappy in her marriage, you may have trouble finding love. If you have struggled with your weight your entire life, there may be some fear about what might happen to you if you were skinny. Having more attention from men can be intimidating and scary when you aren't used to it. The Law of Attraction works, but it is dependent upon you believing that what you want is possible and non-threatening with every ounce of your being—body, mind and spirit.

L: **We all have that inner mean girl who is in full disbelief that she can have a life where her dreams continue to come true. Can you support her with a little science behind your method?**

LR: All the exercises I teach help calm the sympathetic nervous system response, also called a fight-or-flight reaction, so you can get your body and brain more comfortable with taking the steps to change and to grow. One of them, The Easiest Stress Relief Exercise, does this by getting the brain to work bi-laterally. When we are in a sympathetic nervous system response, we switch from bi-lateral to uni-lateral brain function to conserve energy and to utilize our most dominant brain side. When we cross our arms and our legs, then breathe deeply, we send a signal to the body to re-instate bi-lateral brain function, overriding the sympathetic nervous system response physically, causing a relaxation response. When you do this exercise, and think of having what you want, you get your body and brain more comfortable with having it.

While some of the other exercises I teach stimulate points which relate to the Chinese Acupuncture System, by tapping or holding specific points, you can produce some of the same calming effects acupuncturists elicit with your own fingers, without needles! By tapping specific meridian points, as you speak about what is bothering you, you can get your body comfortable with ideas and thoughts that were previously stressful. As you strengthen the meridian system in the face of these stressful thoughts, you can train your body to feel safe having them.

THE SECRET TO MANIFESTING IS LEARNING HOW TO TRAIN YOUR SUBCONSCIOUS MIND AND TO CONDITION YOUR CENTRAL NERVOUS SYSTEM TO BE COMFORTABLE WITH HAVING EVERYTHING YOU DESIRE.

L: **What is one of your juiciest "client miracle manifesting stories" that you can share with the goddesses?**

LR: One of my most recent client stories pops into my head. I had a client join my year-long Believe Boot Camp program when she was out of work, with the understanding that, if she didn't get a job by the end of the first month, she could drop out. Not only did she get a job and stay in the class, four months later she got her dream job! Also, when class started, she hadn't spoken to several members of her family for years due to long standing estrangement. Just last month the entire family got together and had a fun filled reunion. Amazing! And now, after having a dry spell, she is dating. Life partnership is next on our manifesting list. And we are only halfway through the program!

Daily Rituals to Soothe Your Soul (and Mind!)

Exercise Ambien
Do this super relaxing Stress Relief Pose at night for 3-5 minutes when you get into bed; you will most likely fall asleep in it. Doing this nightly, my clients report feeling calmer overall during their days.

This pose helps calm your body's reaction to stress by sending the message to your body to move into a parasympathetic nervous system response, a restive state verses a stress state, so you can have a more peaceful night's sleep.

When you have a fight or flight response to everyday stress, blood rushes from your brain to your limbs to power your escape or fight. When you hold these points, you send a signal to bring blood back to your brain. This reverses the stress response, so you can relax. You are physically conveying the message to your nervous system that, despite the stress you endured during your day, there is no lion chasing you and no gun to your head now, so you can relax and go to sleep. Doing this pose nightly helped me completely alleviate my anxiety during a stressful episode in my life.

Simply place one hand on your forehead and the other across the ridge that runs across the back of your head. Rest your elbows on pillows, so you do not have to hold your arms up and can relax into this position. As you feel pulses in your hands, notice how your body is relaxing.

The Easiest Stress Relief Exercise

This is one of the easiest stress relief exercises I recommend. This exercise can be done to alleviate stress anywhere! I do it on trains, in taxicabs and standing in lines to calm myself down whenever stress strikes. You can't

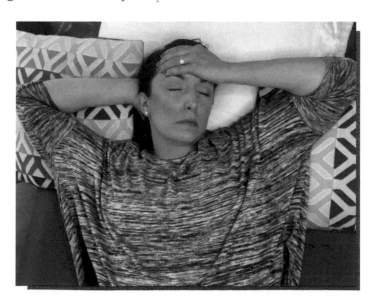

always control what stressors come your way, but with this and the other exercises, you can control how you ultimately react to it.

This particular exercise gets your brain working bilaterally, as explained above. Rate your stress level on a scale of 1-10 before and after doing this exercise, so you can see how this works for you!

Repeating any one of these phrases in this posture is a great way to train your body and central nervous system to be comfortable believing the phrases are possible for you.

I have plenty of time.
I have plenty of money.
I have plenty of help.
I have plenty energy.
I am safe, and prepared.

Simply sit with one ankle crossed over the other. Then, reach your arms out in front of you with the backs of your hands facing one another; cross your arms and clasp your hands together, then place your hands on your lap. Take 3-5 deep breaths, as you repeat one of the mantras above.

ABOUT LARA

Lara Ann Riggio is an expert in Eastern Healing. In her classes, videos and private sessions, she has helped tens of thousands of clients overcome physical aches and pains, emotional resistance to change, stress, anxiety, fatigue and insomnia. Lara's practical, scientific approach to Eastern Healing grounds her work and creates duplicatable results. Lara graduated Summa Cum Laude with a BFA and Dance and a minor in psychology, and she holds advanced certifications from the National Academy of Sports Medicine (CPT and IFS), American Council on Exercise, Muscle Activation Techniques, Eden Energy Medicine, Psych-K, EFT and in Essential Oils. Lara has been featured in The Daily News, Elle, and Women's Day magazines as well as on Fox News, NY1 and the CW11's Morning Show. Lara also contributed the exercise section of the book 100 Questions and Answers about Migraines by Katherine A. Henry, MD and Anthony P. Bossis PhD.

Visit Lara at: http://www.thelaratouch.com ✳

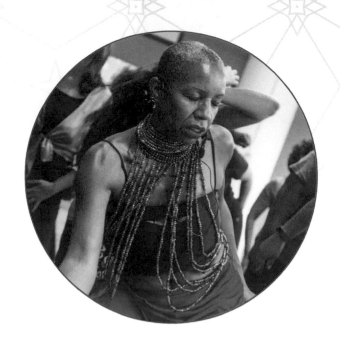

Luscious Movement

———————

VIVE LA FEMME!

Divinely Contributed by

BERNADETTE PLEASANT

Introduction

DURING MY CONTINUOUS RESEARCH OF WHAT IT FEELS LIKE TO COMPLETELY EMBODY the feminine, there was a phrase that kept coming up. It was, "turned on." My head longed to grasp what the hell that meant, and yet my body kept telling me that I sure the hell wasn't going to find it up there!

I had the pleasure of meeting Bernadette Pleasant in a movement class we both were taking. For that entire hour I couldn't keep my eyes off of this gorgeous creature. I know she had to have felt something! It was like watching a movie that you want every young woman to see: This dazzling goddess was *fully in her body—hip circling out messages to the entire group of pure self-acceptance and approval.* Her body can charm a whole fucking room as it moves for her, dazzling her audience, as our souls cry out, "MORE PLEASE!"

Thank Goddess "B" and I clicked, as I deeply desired to one day to be able to know my own body in this way. I began attending every event she put on. The past seven years of working with Bernadette have been a goddess send, as I've been able to release so many stuck emotions from within me that I was terrified to acknowledge. Like most women, I was taught to conceal my deep seated anger and grief. B has inspired me to liberate myself from feeling any shame for having a full range of emotions.

In her Femme!™ class, we move out EVERRYTHANNG from sadness to FLIRTATIOUSNESS! Her one day experience "Emotion In Motion" and her luscious retreat in Jamaica were the revolutionary medicine supporting me in moving out all of the loaded feelings I was carrying after my first year of motherhood. Learning to accept and love the many gorgeous facets of myself has helped me remove the judgment and, instead, set my body on fire! ✳

I DON'T BELIEVE THAT THERE ARE ANY 'GOOD' OR 'BAD' EMOTIONS; JUST EMOTIONS THAT NEED TO BE EXPRESSED.

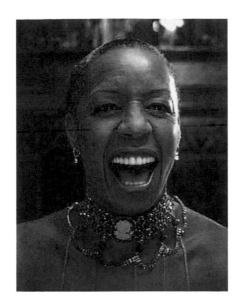

Q&A

WITH BERNADETTE PLEASANT

L: **What was your brilliant inspiration to create a class that has you claim your emotions like rage and lust? I know in our society we have been trained to say "fine" or "good" when others ask us how we are doing. Why do you think it's so difficult for people to pull the mask back and reveal their true feelings?**

B: One of my favorite quotes is from Marianne Williamson, where she says, "Our deepest fear is not that we are inadequate. Our deepest fear is that we are powerful beyond measure. It is our light, not our darkness, that most frightens us. We ask ourselves, Who am I to be brilliant, gorgeous, talented, fabulous? Actually, who are you not to be? Playing small does not serve the world. There is nothing enlightened about shrinking so that other people won't feel insecure around you."

ONCE A WOMAN IS THERE, SHE CAN LEAVE WHAT DOESN'T SERVE HER AND TAKE WITH HER WHATEVER SHE NEEDS.

This is something that women in particular struggle with all the time. In fact, there was a study done at Harvard showing that female students often underperform in classrooms, simply because they shy away from raising their hands as much as their male counterparts. As women, many of us learn to shrink and "play small," to not rock the boat, to not be seen as too much, too sexy or too emotional.

Many of us wind up holding ourselves back from experiencing our own freedom and self-expression. This shows up in so many ways in our bodies and in our lives. That was my inspiration for Femme!™

Femme!™ is actually much more than a movement technique; it's a method of healing. It's a sacred, safe space for women to authentically be themselves, to move in ways that feel good to them, to explore emotions, to release limiting beliefs and to learn to love their bodies, unapologetically!

L: **How have you witnessed this movement liberate healing and support ownership over some of the darker issues we have been trained to suppress?**

B: In Femme!™, much of the work that we do involves honoring the emotions. I don't believe that there are any "good" or "bad" emotions; just emotions that need to be expressed. The Femme!™ Method of Healing uses sensual movement, tribal dance, meditation and other sensory activities to help get a woman out of her head and back into her body.

In a Femme!™ 90-Minute Experience, we take each woman on a journey that includes what we call an "Emotional Tour™." Then, in my full-day workshop (Emotion in Motion), and in my retreats and private client sessions, she gets to take an even deeper dive. I invite women to lose their inhibitions, take up as much space as possible, and to bring all their rage, sadness, fear, lust, joy, whatever they're feeling, to the floor. Once a woman is there, she can leave what doesn't serve her and take with her whatever she needs.

L: **I call you The Queen of "Turn On." Bernadette, what lights your own fire when it comes to Femme!™ and Emotion in Motion?**

B: I love seeing a woman fully in her body, turned on, taking up space, and unapologetically loving herself! It's like being a midwife, birthing that experience for her. I can't even put into words the joy, the pride that I feel. It's truly spiritual; and I get to experience it with her. As I am giving, I am also receiving the Femme!™ Experience. It's orgasmic!

One of my Femme!™-attuned instructors recently described Femme!™ as a method I developed to "alchemize fears, doubts, shame and low self-esteem in a way that reaches in and pulls a woman out, so that she no longer has to hide." I LOVE this description and I especially appreciated the word "alchemize." The sacred science of alchemy isn't about fixing what's wrong. It's about transmuting something already strong, like metal, by drawing out its more brilliant version of itself, like refining gold. That is truly my desire for every woman. It's what Maya Angelou refers to in her poem,

Still I Rise:
Does my sexiness upset you?
Does it come as a surprise?
that I dance like I've got diamonds
at the meeting of my thighs?

THAT . . . is living.

Rituals to Move Through Your Feelings!

Femme!™ isn't just about movement; it's a lifestyle. The Femme!™ way of living is first and foremost about honoring how you feel. And you can do this on a daily basis.

Step One

Take a moment each day. Become aware of your feelings and desires. Whatever crops up—just observe it.

Step Two

Weave in small and large gestures. Learn to refine every moment. Don't just "make do." If you are taking a shower, make it luxurious, take your time, use delicious products that honor your senses, let it be pleasurable. If you've had a busy day, let yourself be indulgent, pour a glass of wine, put your feet up, spend sensual time with your partner and make it magical.

Step Three

Surround yourself with tokens of pleasure to celebrate your love for YOU. Recognize that you are precious and treat yourself to exquisite comfort and pleasure. Don't be okay with ordinary! Instead of that fast food, reward your body with what it really deserves. Don't rush, don't "half ass" your own experiences. I believe in letting everything you do be a sensory experience. Treat yourself to fabrics that feel great on your body, candles that scent the room the way you like, just the right lighting and, of course, music that fits your mood.

Which brings us to . . . Step Four: Movement!

CAN YOU FEEL THE BEAT? What I've found gives a woman the quickest access to emotional release and freedom in her body is the live beat of the drums. Every body responds to the universal, primal call of a drumbeat. It brings out the perfectly wild, childlike, uninhibited side of everyone. I've seen women of all ages, backgrounds and circumstances experience deep healing, primal release, ecstatic pleasure, joy, wonder and self-love! It's like a "time-released" experience; you feel the effects of it while you're in the classroom and then you get to integrate it into the rest of your life, afterward.

WERK! (OR, IN THE ALTERNATIVE: Be as fluid as a stream; light as a feather.) Set aside time each day—even if it's just a few minutes, or, heck, take an hour!—to move in an unrestrained fashion, without thought of who may or may not be watching. Take this time out to move for YOU. To move through whatever you need to express.

MOOD RING (TONE). I believe in having personal playlists that support how you feel. When I feel like I need to get something out, my hard core gangsta rap will be bumping and everyone knows to get out of the way! If I'm feeling deep, earthy and soulful, Nina Simone might be on In the background. Whatever you are feeling—happy, sad, angry, proud, "turned up"—give yourself permission to "have your mood" with a soundtrack that supports how you feel. You can choose to dance, move or do nothing at all. It's your moment. Don't try to shift it. Just be! When I created Femme!™ it was never about dance steps or choreography. It's about moving in a way that feels desirable for you.

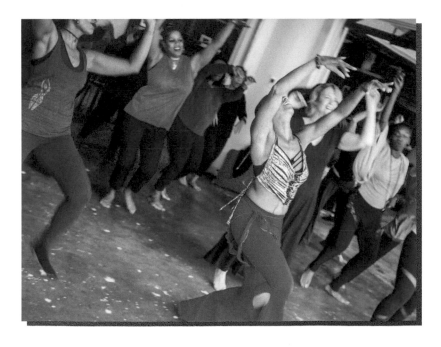

ABOUT BERNADETTE

Bernadette Pleasant has always danced. Her love of music, movement, rhythm and healing comes as naturally to her as breath. She excels at dance and evokes positive reactions in those who watch or dance with her!

When Bernadette first experienced sensual dance, she saw for the first time women move with a flow, grace and emotion that captivated her. The power in their bodies as they moved in expression of how they were feeling in the moment spoke to her, and Bernadette knew that she wanted to both experience movement and express herself with that sort of profound physical and emotional power. Her exploration of sensual dance led her to earn instructor certifications in The Nia Technique®, Nia® 5 Stages, Ageless Grace® and Pole dance. She also studied African, Tribal and Free Dance and began integrating and infusing these dance forms with sensuality, visualization, meditations, affirmations and techniques from the healing arts to create Femme!™. She is also certified in Integrated Energy Therapy.

In the Femme!™ Experience, Bernadette creates a safe space for women of all ages, backgrounds, body types and dance skills to explore their sensual selves. Women are empowered to fully embrace and embody all of their emotions and fully express them through movement; joy, sorrow, rage, ecstasy and more are all welcome at Femme!™. In Femme!™ women are infused with the affirmation, "It's your body; you can do whatever you want with it—including love it unapologetically!"

Visit Bernadette at: www.livefemme.com ✳

"

THE SACRED
SCIENCE OF
ALCHEMY ISN'T
ABOUT FIXING
WHAT'S WRONG.
IT'S ABOUT
TRANSMUTING
SOMETHING
ALREADY
STRONG ...

3

VIBRANT & GORGEOUS HEALTH

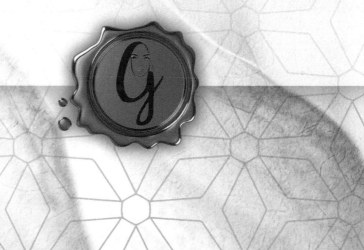

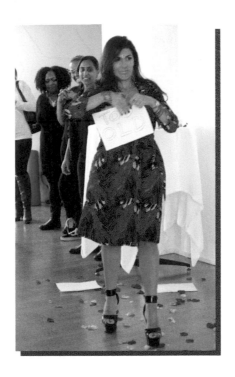

I WAS TAUGHT, LIKE MOST WOMEN, TO PICK APART EVERY SQUARE INCH OF MY BODY. It began with conversations with myself and then transitioned to unsolicited comments about my body from others like, "You're way too skinny! A little underdeveloped there? You're 13, where are your tits?" As I became an adult, the comments evolved to, "Oh my! You have put on so much weight!" and, "Damn, look at that ass!" And when I was pregnant: "Are you sure you aren't having twins?" After the baby, "Wow! You've lost SO much weight!"

Why has the world sent out this message that it's normal for women to body obsess? Why do strangers and friends feel it's okay to consistently comment on our bodies, yet we feel ashamed to speak up, as if we are being "impolite"? Why can't women put their "nice" aside and truthfully say how that really makes us feel.

In my 39 years of life, I have been visited by every body label from the "too skinny girl" to the "very thick girl." Even the "You've lost so much weight!" feels like a punch to the gut. Why can't we just give women authentic compliments like, "You look amazing"?!

WE HAVE GOT IT ALL WRONG— GIVING THE SCALE A KEY TO OUR HAPPINESS. FUCK THAT!

My story with body shame began at age seven, when I was put on the drug Ritalin for my supposed "hyper-activeness." Unbeknownst to me, it was an appetite suppressant, in addition to being a substance made to zone people out of their feelings. The moment I popped that pill I would instantly feel full. I took one pill at breakfast and one before lunchtime. By the time I came home from school, I would be famished from not eating the first two meals of the day.

Let me tell you, *honey*! I bragged about being able to put down an entire large pizza, a carton of Oreos, and a pint of ice cream without blinking. The other thing that happened was I couldn't gain a pound. I was the skinny girl at school, and by the time I was in 6th grade, and all of the other girls were wearing bras, there I stood underdeveloped as ever. Of course, I was teased with names, called "flat chested," and warned that I'd better stuff my bra if I wanted boys to be interested in me!

Unfortunately, this stage lasted all the way through junior high. It wasn't until I was actually taken off of Ritalin during the summer going into 9th grade that I began to develop any semblance of a teenage body. And then—BOOM! I walked into 9th grade with the curves of a grown-ass woman. Suddenly, I found myself the center of many teenage boys' and older men's attention. It was overwhelming. I had mixed feelings of being flattered to be in this spotlight and yet having no idea what to do with all of this.

The attention became too much, and because I was used to eating doughnuts, cookies, and fast food without gaining an ounce, there was no reason to abandon any of that. By the end of 9th grade, I could no longer fit into any resemblance of a skinny jean.

I now had to transform into the "big girl" and use name-brand clothing and humor to keep being "liked."

My first episode of binge eating was at my aunt's wedding in California. I was 15. The crème brûlée was SO good that I think I ate about 2 ½ before my belly let me know it wasn't feeling too good. I was terrified about gaining weight from the richness of all that dessert. It felt like enough pressure that my "skinny" outfit was too tight, so I snuck off into a bathroom stall and stuck my finger down my throat. Hoping no one would hear me.

I can still see that moment in my mind. A deep darkness took over my body that I can't put into words. It was as if I began carrying a horrible secret that I could never allow anyone to find out about. This became the norm every time I ate too much.

SUDDENLY, I FOUND MYSELF
THE CENTER OF MANY TEENAGE
BOYS' AND OLDER MEN'S ATTENTION.
IT WAS OVERWHELMING. THERE
WERE MIXED FEELINGS OF
BEING FLATTERED TO BE
IN THIS SPOTLIGHT AND YET
HAVING NO IDEA WHAT TO DO
WITH ALL OF THIS.

After high school, I became obsessed with diets. I tried everything from herbal laxative teas (that always sent me running for a bathroom at the most inconvenient times) to Jenny Craig. None of these "diets" seemed to help heal the underlying old beliefs I had about myself.

By age 27, I was totally addicted to processed sugars, needed to down at least three Red Bulls a day in order to have *any* type of energy, and was consuming frozen, boxed food for time-saving meals.

At a time when I had become so resigned to my body "fate" that I was eating about 15 pieces of milk chocolate wrapped up in little kiss wrappers, my dear friend Cathy Vignola was sent into my life! Cathy happened to be going to the Integrative Institute of Nutrition in NYC. One day, while having a casual hangout, I shared with her my food woes and the struggle I was having with my body. She suggested I start by switching over my fruits and vegetables to organic and noticing if my body felt any different. Oh goddess did it! Suddenly, I was turned on by the sweetness of an apple, and I found myself craving homemade smoothies and fresh salads full of colorful veggies. There was no bad taste left in my mouth as if they had been drenched in chemical pesticides! And with the genius switch to organic food *my fuzzy thinking became clear. BOOM!*

WE HAVE GOT IT ALL WRONG— GIVING THE SCALE A KEY TO OUR HAPPINESS.

But my obsession with food and my body was far from over. On an evening out, one of the goddesses in my circle could feel my nervous energy while ordering dinner. The advice she gave me was GOLDEN! She pointed out that, if we are holding onto any *guilt* around food, just that alone can hold weight in the body. Her suggestion was to slow down, eat for my own PLEASURE, and savor each yummy bite without a thread of judgment.

I started to see the obsession dissipating. Her words resonated with me on a cellular level. Shortly after that I took a deep, audacious

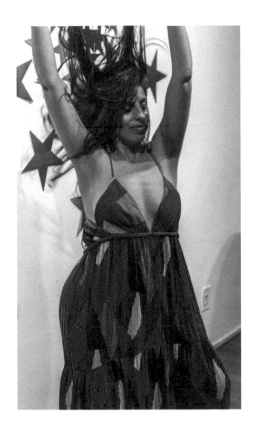

breath and set my scale out to the curb for the garbage man to haul away forever. There would be no more mornings where the number on the scale determined the way my day went. HELL TO THE NO! A long awaited acceptance settled into my soul. I realized that, for the rest of my life, my body's weight will fluctuate, and I am at total peace with that. It was time to LOVE each and every curve that the goddess has blessed me with.

NO! A long awaited acceptance settled into my soul. I realized that, for the rest of my life, my body's weight will fluctuate, and I am at total peace with that. For the first time in a long while I wasn't tasting chemicals or pesticides when I ate my fruits and veggies!

In 2014, after not eating meat for over 10 years, my body woke up one day pregnant with a little one growing in my belly AND a deep craving for animal protein. I had been a vegan the year before for six months. Suddenly, my menu was full of grass-fed burgers, steaks, and organic eggs. I craved this day in and day out for those nine months. After six months of breastfeeding, my desires shifted once again to more greens, fish, and some sort of weekly red meat.

My metabolism has soared the highest I can remember since I was 13. It has to be from continuous breastfeeding and chasing after an Aries growing toddler! After watching "What The Health," I'm back to vegan.

I'm sharing my story to let you know, goddesses, that I am SO, SO far from perfect with my health. I have learned to love my voluptuous body, and I eat for pure pleasure now, nothing else will do. I worship my own body with total approval. But don't get me wrong—my love for the occasional French Fries and red velvet cake is here to STAY!

I'm inspired to turn you on to what I've learned, and I'm EXCITED for you to feel empowered around your own health, too, Beauties—so let's DO THIS together! These next experts are going to lead you into a brand new relationship with your health and give you amazing tools along your journey. ✳

"

A LONG AWAITED
ACCEPTANCE SETTLED
INTO MY SOUL. I
REALIZED THAT, FOR
THE REST OF MY LIFE,
MY BODY'S WEIGHT
WILL FLUCTUATE,
AND I AM AT TOTAL
PEACE WITH THAT. IT
WAS TIME TO LOVE
EACH AND EVERY
CURVE THAT THE
GODDESS HAS BLESSED
ME WITH.

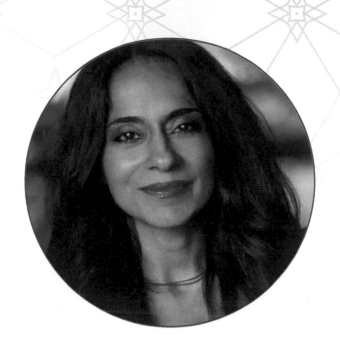

Health

ENJOY
THE SILENCE

✳

Divinely Contributed by

DR. KARUNA SABNANI

Introduction

LIVING IN A WORLD WHERE WE ARE
CONSISTENTLY BEING BOMBARDED WITH
messages about the "right ways to eat or exercise," many health
experts miss the mark regarding what comes *before*. Truth talking
here: When you are running from one meeting to the next without
taking a pause, forgetting to eat, and only getting three to four hours
of sleep, something is off. You have stopped listening to that voice
inside that is screaming SLOW DOWN! It's possible you threw your
relationship with balance out the door. How can you even decipher
whether to choose a decadent, healthy meal over a greasy ass slice
of pizza?!

A body running on fumes can do no good for the Goddess! I had
the pleasure of discussing this with Dr. Karuna Sabnani. Her genius
philosophy is all about simplicity. She has discovered ways to bring
self-care and healthy tools to goddesses on the go who have super
full lives. This was exactly what I desired for her to share with you! Our
bodies are made for and require exquisite care. Immerse yourselves
in some of her glorious goodness and dive into the time-saving rituals
she created below. ✳

"

... I EXPERIENCED
A BACK INJURY
THAT HELPED ME
RECOGNIZE HOLES
IN THE MEDICAL
SYSTEM, AND I FELT
THIS INNER URGE TO
DO IT DIFFERENTLY,
TO REALLY LISTEN
TO OTHERS AND TO
GIVE THEM, IN TURN,
TOOLS TO BRING OUT
THEIR TRUE VOICES.

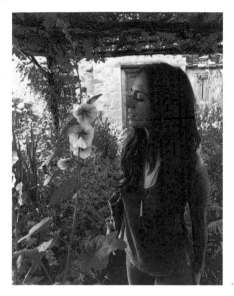

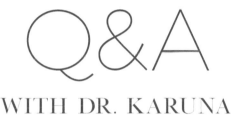

WITH DR. KARUNA

L: **Can you share a little about your own personal story? What sparked your passion for helping women find that delicate balance between overworking and having a healthy lifestyle?**

DK: I grew up in the United States as a first generation girl of Indian descent and the oldest of three children. There is a lot of suppression of women in my culture. My mother told me a story when I was seven years old about how my grandma would not let her go to medical school because "no man wanted to marry a woman smarter than him."

This story impacted me so deeply that I still remember telling my childhood best friend that, one day, I would grow up and help women to be free. I went on to attend Mount Holyoke College, the first women's college in the U.S.A, because, at that time, "Harvard wasn't admitting women." In college, I saw firsthand the way women harm themselves by depriving their bodies of nourishment, both through food and intimacy, in order to keep a certain image. This left a deep impression on me, as I saw gorgeous and brilliant women self-abuse rather than love themselves.

Additionally, I experienced a back injury that helped me recognize holes in the medical system, and I felt this inner urge to do it differently, to really listen to others and to give them, in turn, tools to bring out their true voices.

IN COLLEGE, I SAW FIRSTHAND THE WAY WOMEN HARM THEMSELVES BY DEPRIVING THEIR BODIES OF NOURISHMENT, BOTH THROUGH FOOD AND INTIMACY, IN ORDER TO KEEP A CERTAIN IMAGE.

L: **Why do you think women have gotten into this debilitating pattern of ignoring, and even suppressing, the messages our bodies consistently send us?**

DK: I think that society has a contorted view of what true power is in America. Our values are off. Silence and a slow pace are associated with being "second best." With technology speeding up at its current pace, society feels that *the push faster, more, quicker mentality is correct.*

In actuality, being like water, fluid and mutable, is authentic power. This is the power a woman innately has, but the messages from advertisements and city living drown it out for most. There is a sense I hear often of being left behind or being less than if certain outer achievement marks aren't attained. Focusing so much on the outer has many women not only starving to hear their inner voices but also depleted physically due to body image myths.

L: **If there was one ritual you could shout from the mountain tops, what would that be?**

DK: To take between 5 and 30 minutes every morning and every night for yourself—to start the day fresh and then release the day before sleeping. I call this creating "bookends." This means no computer or electronics during this time. Instead, do your meditation practice and give time to Silence. Check in with your whispers (inner voice) before the day drowns them out; and at night, let it all go. I can't emphasis this ritual enough.

Health Ritual: TDD Relaxation Massage

What is Time Deficit Disorder (TDD)?

You are a multi-tasking connoisseur. Elevator reflections and vanity mirrors in your car serve as your dressing room. You skip meals. You use lunch break to complete deliverables. You forget to drink water. You gulp down meals. You eat standing up. You live for on-the-go options. The term "New York Minute" was created for you! Your magic genie wish is for more hours in the day, and you groan at your email inbox.

You have a codependent relationship with your cell phone: It is your alarm clock; the first thing you reach for in the morning and the last thing you let go of at night. You text with one finger on the treadmill or while getting a manicure. "Siri" is your closest friend (yes, the truth hurts), and "Busy" is your middle name. You create early bed times for your kids just so you can clean the house, breathe and eat dinner . . . at midnight. You work three jobs.

CHECK IN WITH YOUR WHISPERS (INNER VOICE) BEFORE THE DAY DROWNS THEM OUT.

You dream about sleep, and you are scheduled down to the minute—there is no room for the unexpected. Regular workouts, diets and relaxation routines feel like "big" commitments. Overwhelmed, you choose nothing. The irony of it all? Relaxation itself stresses you out.

If you are reading this, the odds are great that your life often feels like a non-stop emergency. Until you can retire to a cave in the Himalayas—or choose to slow down, you need to learn tricks so that not only every minute counts, but also adds value to your life. Developing proper systems can help to create relaxation in all your rushed moments. You may be in the rat race, but you don't have to *be* a rat!

Daily attention to stress reduction is the secret to health and life enjoyment. Pay attention to these essentials. To get relief, self-prescribe a "dream" or "time-deficit" (TDD) de-stress dosage that works for your schedule.

A "dream dosage" is for when you have more time. This should be the goal. The TDD dosage is for when you are in a time crunch. Your de-stress dosage will turn from minutes to hours, and through daily practice will become a habit.

DREAM DOSAGE: Healthy touch is indispensable and whisks away tension like nothing else. Get professional full-body massages or trade massages with a loved one. Learn to give yourself self-massage. Experiment with different styles of massage and choose what relaxes you the most.

TIME DEFICIT DOSAGE: Massage your scalp and feet. Scalp: Use your fingers or a scalp massager. The head holds a lot of tension, and when released, is pleasure you will want to repeat. Feet: Use a little lotion and massage them before bed. Both of these techniques will improve sleep as well. Massage for 1-5 minutes.

TDD RELAXATION MASSAGE OIL RECIPE:
(The smell alone will relax you!)

SUPPLIES:
1 ounce of Sweet Almond Oil or Grapeseed Oil
15 drops of Lavender oil
15 drops of Ylang Ylang oil

DIRECTIONS:
Pour the 1 ounce bottle of oil into a bowl. Add the essential oils and stir. Pour the oils into a dark one-ounce glass bottle. Store in the refrigerator.

HEALTHY TOUCH EQUALS
PLEASURE & RELAXATION

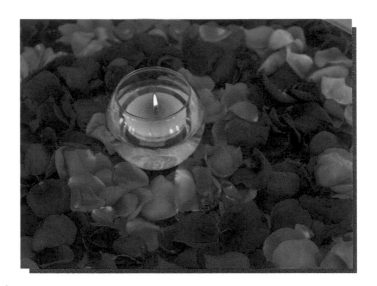

ABOUT KARUNA

Dr. Karuna Sabnani's knowledge of health and inner & outer beauty is vast, which has made her one of the leading experts sought out by the Huffington Post. She was also the personal naturopathic expert for supermodel IMAN's company IMAN Cosmetics. She has made appearances on national networks, and has been featured on The Dr. OZ Show and actress Judy Greer's show Reluctantly Healthy on The CW Network.

Dr. Karuna teaches the importance of slowing down to enjoy life with ease and beauty, while helping women detox from old habits, food, household and beauty products that may harm their bodies. As a woman, she understands what our bodies are constantly going through. Her on-the-go advice for us is time-saving and supports women in being spiritually centered.

Visit Dr. Karuna at: www.karunanaturopathic.com ✳

"

... TAKE BETWEEN
5 AND 30 MINUTES
EVERY MORNING
AND EVERY NIGHT
FOR YOURSELF
... START THE
DAY FRESH AND
THEN RELEASE
THE DAY BEFORE
SLEEPING. I CALL
THIS CREATING
'BOOKENDS.'

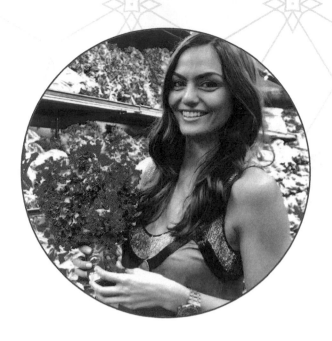

Health

BEAUTIFUL
FOOD

Divinely Contributed by

MARIA MARLOWE

Introduction

I MET MARIA ABOUT SEVEN YEARS AGO ON
A PHOTO SHOOT FOR L'OREAL. WE WERE
both in our previous, what you would call, "fabulous" careers. I was the
makeup artist and Maria was the model. But were we sitting around
dishing on the latest celebrity crush or beauty craze? NO, GODDESSES,
NOOOO! We discovered that we share a love for kale, raw chocolate,
and avocado. Organic, raw, vegan food was the "thing" back then.
Together, we shared notes on our favorite vegan meals, how green
juice had given us liiiifeeee, and the best *raw* restaurants NYC had to
offer. The first tIme Maria came over, she surprised our goddess circle
with this ah-mazing, homemade raw chocolate dessert that I
still fantasize about!

A year later, I found out that Maria had gone after her dream of
becoming a health coach! Her belief is that food can be medicine for
our bodies, especially when we can't understand why we are having a
pesky breakout. She has helped many of her ladies get their goddess
glow back by looking at how the foods they are eating and their hectic
lifestyles may be the real culprits. Mmmmhmmm, yes ladies, you may
want to put down that piece of brie! One way she says to love your

body is by loving the foods you ingest. But that doesn't mean your days have to be blasé! Just the opposite is true. Maria encourages her clients to indulge in having a kick-ass social life rather than isolating yourself because you are "eating healthy." Dive in below with some of Maria's body-loving rituals to find out how! ✳

I USED TO THINK THAT GOING ON A DIET MEANT PEELING THE FRIED COATING OFF MY CHICKEN NUGGETS. SERIOUSLY.

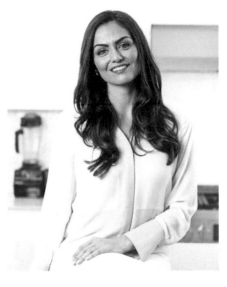

Q&A

WITH MARIA MARLOWE

L: **How has social media skewed our view of what a real woman's body is? Where do you see this affecting our level of self-confidence?**

M: We are constantly bombarded with images of the "ideal woman" in magazines, on TV, and even Instagram. Typically, our first inclination is to compare ourselves to these women, and when our physique or face or hair isn't a mirror image of that person, who we have decided is the standard of ultimate beauty, we then start feeling bad about ourselves. We look in the mirror and tell ourselves how fat and ugly and disgusting we are, and then are surprised when we keep self-sabotaging and remain heavier than we'd like, or unhappy. Words are everything. They shape your life, they shape your body.

The first step to losing weight is not diet or exercise. It is changing your belief system. Shifting your perspective to look at your body in reverence and awe. To be grateful that you woke up this morning, that you have strong legs to take you where you want to go, sparkling eyes to see the beautiful world, and strong arms to hug the ones you love. Only when you look in the mirror and love yourself will you achieve your health and wellness goals.

WORDS ARE EVERYTHING. THEY SHAPE YOUR LIFE, THEY SHAPE YOUR BODY.

L: **Maria, you are known for being a health fairy in the kitchen with your mouth watering recipes! So many of us don't want to give up our hearty dishes, yet desire to feel healthy. What are your two favorite dishes you have transformed into delish?**

M: I love coming up with healthier versions of traditional comfort foods. My favorite is a cashew cream cake that tastes just like creamy Italian cheesecake, but is made solely with fruit and nuts. It is divine. I also love my "mac and cheese," where I top brown rice pasta with a sweet potato, non-dairy cream sauce that will blow your mind. When you make your meals out of whole ingredients, you never have to worry about overeating, because you automatically feel full and satisfied on just the right amount of food.

L: **What is the one food you can't live without? We all have that one thing we can't walk past without having a tiny bite. I have been known to wake up craving Red Velvet Cake and French Fries.**

M: I know you're hoping I would say deep fried Oreos or something, but I honestly can't live without dark, leafy greens. I crave them. I eat spinach salad for breakfast sometimes. I have literally rewired my taste buds to only crave the foods that absolutely nourish my body. I never feel like I'm deprived, and whenever I want something, I eat it . . . it's just that I no longer ever have a desire for cookies and cakes and foods that don't ultimately serve my body. My once-in-a-while guilty pleasure, though, is organic corn tortilla chips. And I may or may not eat more coconut sugar-sweetened dark chocolate than is necessary.

Health Rituals

Daily Health Ritual
One way to start eliminating negative self talk, and learn to love your body, is to dry brush while doing positive affirmations. Every morning when you wake up, take about 5 minutes to dry brush in front of the mirror, stark naked. As you go over each body part, say out loud all

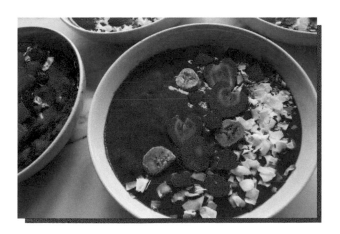

the things you love or are grateful for about that specific part, or your body in general. When a negative thought pops up, immediately bite your tongue and replace it with two nice things.

Step by step action for long term success

For something we typically do at least 3 times a day, most of us have no clue how the food we eat affects our bodies. That it could be the culprit behind our breakouts, our low energy, our migraines, and even our cancer risk, is a concept foreign to many. I'm here to change that. As a girl who struggled with her weight and was covered in acne and perpetually sick, I used to think that going on a diet meant peeling the fried coating off my chicken nuggets. Seriously.

THERE ARE CERTAIN LAWS OF NATURE, AND IF YOU PUT JUNK INTO YOUR BODY, IT WILL BREAK DOWN AT SOME POINT.

For the past 10 years, I have since dedicated my life to food and nutrition, drawing the connection between our ailments and our diets. I now teach people how to decipher their digestive issues, weight that won't budge, low energy, and acne, because I know how frustrating it is to be at war with your body. It's our right to know how food affects our bodies, and our duty to take care of ourselves. When we are in peak form, we are able to best serve the ones we love. Here are some ideas for leading a healthier lifestyle, and loving it:

Change your language

The first step in losing weight or improving your health is mindset. When you see your body as a gorgeous, glittering temple, all of a sudden, you want to choose the healthiest foods and move your body often. Replace the broken record of negative thoughts in your head with gratitude for your always gorgeous, no-matter-what-size-it-is body. If you want to lose weight, acknowledge how beautiful your body is now, and that it's a work in progress to get to your ideal. You may have fat, but you are not fat. Switch your language. Repeat the mantra—"I treat my body like gold."

When someone makes fun of you for ordering a salad

Remember that, at the end of the day, it's your body, not theirs, and you're the only one who will have to deal with the consequences of making food choices that are not right for you, whether that is bloating and gas, low energy, not fitting into anything, or getting a scary diagnosis.

There are certain laws of nature, and if you put junk into your body, it will break down at some point. Be strong in your resolve and know why you are choosing a healthy dish—because you love yourself so much, you would never desecrate the sacred temple that is your body. Remind them you're not restricting yourself or feeling deprived, but that you truly desire the healthy dish you chose.

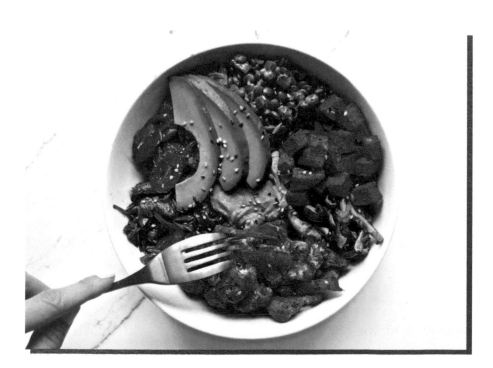

If you have "No Time" to Eat Healthy

Remember that time is the only even playing field we have. Everyone has 24 hours in a day. It is your priorities that determine what you do with those hours. When you commit to loving yourself and putting your health first, you will *make time* to grocery shop, cook, and work out, and make it a point to order healthy and do the best you can in every situation.

ABOUT MARIA

Maria Marlowe's holistic (not hippie) approach to health has helped hundreds of women and men lose weight, embrace healthy eating, and feel better in their bodies. Having experienced weight and skin problems first-hand, she intimately understands that weight loss is about more than just food and calories, and flawless skin is about more than just expensive creams. Both require an understanding of the food-body connection, a detailed road map for replacing bad habits, and in a sense, re-learning not just what to eat, but how to think. From eliminating excuses, to improving self-confidence, to dealing with the emotional eating triggers, Maria has the ability to laser in on what's keeping her clients from their ideal bodies.

To date, Maria has worked with many celebrities and has appeared on The Dr. Oz Show, NBC, and CBS. She has been featured in InStyle, Vogue, The New York Times, Well+Good NYC and many more.

Maria graduated summa cum laude from Fordham University, studied holistic nutrition at The Institute for Integrative Nutrition and plant-based cooking at The Natural Gourmet Institute. She lives and works in New York City.

Visit Maria at: www.mariamarlowe.com ✳

"

THE FIRST STEP
TO LOSING
WEIGHT IS NOT
DIET OR EXERCISE.
IT IS CHANGING
YOUR BELIEF
SYSTEM.

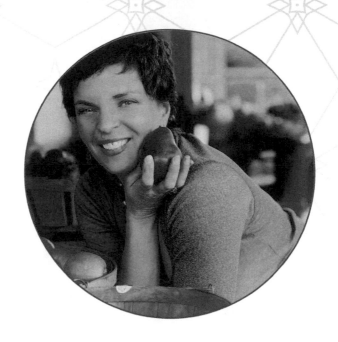

Health

FORGIVING YOUR CORE WOUND

✳

Divinely Contributed by

MARCELLA FRIEL

Introduction

WE OFTEN OVERLOOK HOW MUCH FOOD IS TIED TO EMOTIONS. MANY OF OUR EARLIEST memories include celebrations with plates and dishes of our favorite food, which we then associated with joy. Personally, the moments when my family was consumed with food were the most peaceful. Often I would find myself impulsively eating, believing that there wasn't enough food for every member in my household. I began to hoard food, creating a false belief (that felt so true) that I would starve if I didn't. This continued on into my thirties, as I tried to numb out the feelings I was too scared to deal with. I found myself at social events, filling my plate up, going back for seconds and thirds, and eating until my belly couldn't take it anymore. *I would leave these occasions that were supposed to be full of happiness with an extreme dose of sadness and shame instead.*

Many of us feel hopeless when it comes to our eating addictions. Often we have to go deep down into our emotional well to heal this part of ourselves. I wanted to bring in someone who's an expert at helping women repair their fixations with food, and Marcella Friel is dynamic at revealing what's been at the source of her clients' eating habits. ✳

One of my favorite stories of Marcella's is about a client who was addicted to diet soda and couldn't seem to let it go. Marcella first helped her client identify the craving. She then used an energy technique to cure this urge to reach for a soda. Years later? *This client hasn't experienced a single day with the desire for a diet soda since then.* Goddesses, my deepest wish is that you get some relief and new tools when these old habits with food come up. Marcella's ritual will help you let go of some of the old energetic charge.

HOW DOES FORGIVENESS PLAY INTO THIS? IN OH, SO MANY WAYS.

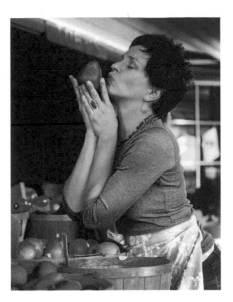

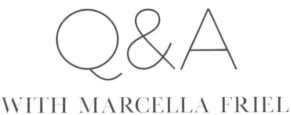

WITH MARCELLA FRIEL

———————

L: **Marcella, why do you think self-forgiveness is so important in healing those patterns with food that we have not been able to conquer?**

M: My clients are women who know their issues with food are not about the food. They're women who have been yo-yo dieting their whole lives or whose mothers put them on a diet when they were eight years old. They've been so obsessed with their food and body image struggles that they can't imagine it could ever change—although some part of them can imagine it, and that's why they contact me.

THE TRANSFORMATIONAL PROCESS IS NOT EASY. IF A CLIENT CAN LOVE HERSELF ENOUGH TO STICK WITH IT THROUGH THE UNCOMFORTABLE SPOTS, ALL SORTS OF MIRACLES START TO HAPPEN.

How does forgiveness play into this? In oh, so many ways. Physiologically, forgiveness reduces the chronic inflammation associated with stressful emotions, which then allows a woman's body to relax and *let go* of the weight rather than struggle to *lose* the weight. Can you feel the difference in that? Forgiveness also empowers a woman to make more self-loving choices in every area of her life, including but not limited to her relationship with self-nourishment.

L: **What is the most common emotional hold you see women challenged with when it comes to food?**

M: Self-blame is by far, hands down, the biggest emotional obstacle to body love for women. We blame ourselves for not looking like Barbie dolls or for not getting a bikini body in 30 days. Because we are vessels by nature, we absorb and hold all the shaming messages fed to us by society and our families. I believe that unconditional self-love and self-acceptance is the way out of the struggle.

I had a client who became a nervous wreck every time she went out to lunch with her girlfriends. She was so anxious over what she should and shouldn't order from the menu. I drilled down to the core belief driving her behavior, which was: "Everybody else gets to have fun but me." After we cleared that belief in a few EFT sessions, she lost 15 pounds without even trying and felt totally comfortable ordering whatever she wanted. This is what I love about my work. I see miracles like that happening all the time!

L: **How do you help women relieve their obsession with food and reignite their confidence around life?**

M: I help women understand the wisdom of their struggles. There's some way the soul is trying to protect itself against further harm. The transformational process is not easy. If a client can love herself enough to stick with it through the uncomfortable spots, all sorts of miracles start to happen. She loses a few pounds without trying. She gets up to walk first thing in the morning. She begins her day with a nourishing breakfast. Most importantly, she builds an unshakable foundation of self-love that stays true through any challenge. That's what I call the Gift of the Goddess.

Health Ritual: The Decision to Forgive

Forgiveness is the key to all healing. And forgiveness begins with a decision. This ritual is about the decision to forgive. You might or might not yet experience forgiveness through this ritual, but you will be setting the stage for forgiveness to come to you, be it suddenly or gradually. Take it on as a daily practice if necessary.

You'll need a mirror, a candle, and a journal. You'll also need a private space free from interruption.

Plan to spend at least 30 minutes performing this ritual.

Light your candle.

Begin by sitting in meditation with your eyes closed and your hands on your heart, connecting to your heartbeat. If your attention wanders, bring it back to that beating heart. Sit this way until you feel more settled in your awareness.

Think about who you want to forgive, whether yourself or someone else. Spend a few minutes journaling about why you want to forgive this person. If it feels hard to forgive, write about that.

When you are complete with writing, look at yourself in the mirror. Say aloud, "[Name], I have decided to forgive you, as best I can."

Repeat this aloud until you feel complete, then spend a few moments being present to the thoughts and feelings that arise. Write them down if necessary.

Repeat this practice until the forgiveness feels complete.

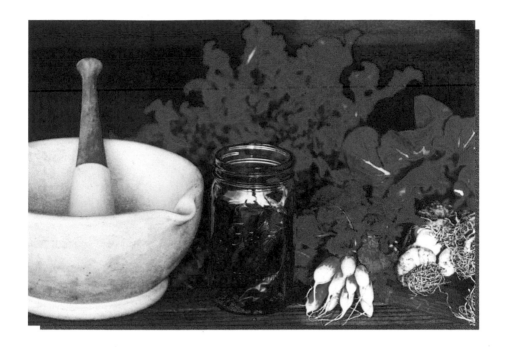

ABOUT MARCELLA

Having cooked and taught in meditation retreat centers across North America, Marcella Friel runs Tapping with Marcella, a food and body image coaching practice that supports health-conscious women in loving and forgiving themselves, their food and their figure.

Marcella teaches mindful eating retreats across the United States, and her writing has been featured in the Shambhala Times, Elephant Journal, and elsewhere.

A longtime meditation practitioner, Marcella combines laser-sharp insight, playful humor, and gentle inquisitiveness to help clients feel held, seen, and at ease as she helps them release their negative core beliefs about themselves and their food.

Visit Marcella at: www.tappingwithmarcella.com ✳

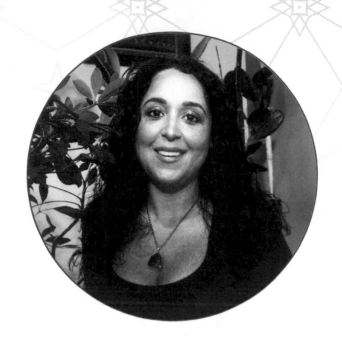

Health

DELICIOUS & WHOLESOME

∗

Divinely Contributed by

IBETLIZA FRIAS

Introduction

AS A YOUNG GIRL, I GREW UP IN A HOUSEHOLD WHERE WE WERE CONSTANTLY warned that all the "good food" was going to run out, resulting in me learning to become a speed eater. I was damn proud of how fast I could down a box of Twinkies! I never realized that so much of this was tied to a feeling of survival. When I was in my 20's I started to have digestive problems, stuffing myself to the point that the food in my belly would come right back up. Acid reflux, anyone? Gassiness? Yes! Ugh! I couldn't seem to figure this one out on my own. When it came to eating healthy, I was resigned to believing that nothing would ever change. Thank Goddess Ibetliza came into my life when I really needed to try something new around food.

The first thing Ibetliza guided me into was *slowing down*—pumping the brakes on "how fast" I could devour a sweet potato fry. Instead, I began to leisurely savor each bite with absolute pleasure. Ibetliza totally boosted my cooking experience with her bowl-licking recipes. Talk about a party in your mouth! *Eating healthy could actually be decadent instead of tasting like a piece of grass wrapped in cardboard?!* This goddess in the kitchen believes in turning on ALL of your senses and using your intuition, so that cooking and eating are freeing experiences. ✳

There'll be no more following rigid recipes now, my loves! It's time to break some rules!

Hold on tight to your taste buds. It's time for fun and pleasure to take the lead in your mind, body and kitchen!

ONE OF MY FAVORITE THINGS TO DO IS TEACH WOMEN TO TAP INTO THEIR INTUITION WHILE COOKING.

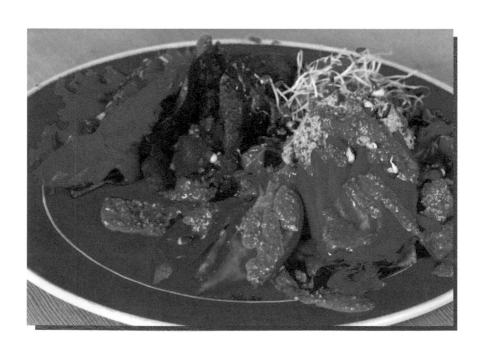

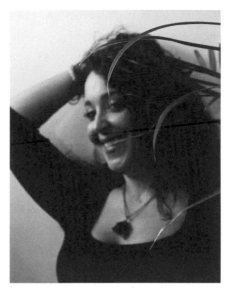

Q&A

WITH IBETLIZA FRIAS

————

L: **Ibetliza, so many women walk into the kitchen and feel completely overwhelmed! They have no idea where to begin and feel pressured to cook a meal that takes hours and endless ingredients. How can we bring some pleasure and delight into this first step?**

I: That's a great question, Leora. What I would start with is creating this to be an experience instead of another dreadful chore or thing to do. The energy we bring to our food is so important. You want to set the mood/intention for your meal. What I suggest is, playing some of your favorite music (feel free to have a spontaneous dance party while your water is boiling!), light a candle, and give a moment of thanks for having time with yourself.

L: **It's easy for me to cook out of habit; I'm sure most women feel safe cooking what we know. After a while it starts to feel automatic, which takes away from the fun. How do you consistently stay inspired to create these fabulous dishes?**

I: I grew up on my mother's Dominican cooking, and I actually come from a family of cooks. I watched my family cook with the typical Hispanic-American seasonings that weren't really healthy for me. That's when I started to explore cooking with more natural spices and noticed how delicious and fulfilling my meals were becoming as a result.

   I teach women to take the lid off of what it means to eat healthy, yummy food. I love playing with different flavors. For example: Salads never have to have the same dressings, and collard greens can be cooked Southern or with an Asian-influence.

L: **So many of us get caught up following a recipe to the freakin' tee, which feels rigid. What is your take on that?**

I: One of my favorite things to do is teach women to tap into their intuition while cooking. Each one of us has a unique palette. Some of us like it spicy, sweeter, or light-mild. The more you let go of the rules and make room for fun and play, the more your confidence builds and you're guided by your own creativity.

Health Ritual: Creating Two Meals and Dessert—Simple & Delicious!

GODDESS BLEND

Berry-Infused Breakfast Smoothie for a Goddess On The Go! This delicious breakfast smoothie is the perfect Goddess blend for a boost of morning energy. No need to miss your coffee with this one. The handfuls of spinach will do the trick to wake you up effortlessly, not to mention the natural sweetness of your favorite berries will add the morning comfort you are looking for. It is a full and complete meal, as the protein from the almond milk will be sure to keep you satisfied. You will be sooo ready to take on your day!

INGREDIENTS:

3 handfuls of organic baby spinach

1 cup of unsweetened almond milk

½ cup of water

1½ cups of your favorite frozen berries

⅛ tsp of vanilla extract

½ inch of fresh ginger root

2 packets of Truvia

3 dashes of cinnamon

DIRECTIONS:

Blend together in a bullet or a regular store blender. Serve in your favorite tall wine glass!

COMFORT POT PIE

Vegetable, gluten-free pot pie. Who would've thought comfort food could come with all of these health benefits? Omit any guilt associated with "comfort" food—this one meal holds a wealth of deliciousness from a load of root veggies. Not only will it satisfy your hunger, but also your sugar cravings from all the natural sugar in the vegetables, so you'll kick that sweet tooth to the curb with this super easy-to-make dish!

INGREDIENTS:

1 head of organic cauliflower
1 cup diced celery, 1 cup diced carrots, 1 cup diced onions, 1 cup diced sweet potatoes, 1 cup diced yams, 3 cloves garlic—you guessed it—diced!
Dry oregano and basil to taste
Sea salt & pepper to taste
1 tsp of Braggs Amino Acid sauce
1 Tbsp of coconut oil
Garlic powder to taste
⅛ cup almond milk
2 Tbsp finely chopped chives
3 dashes of turmeric

DIRECTIONS:

Sauté in pan all of your root veggies (minus the cauliflower) with dry herbs, salt and pepper in the coconut oil, and cook till tender.

Make cauliflower mashed potatoes by boiling a head of cauliflower, broken into florets, in water and sea salt for 15 minutes. Once stems are soft, blend the cauliflower in a food processor with organic butter or coconut oil and 3 dashes of turmeric. This will give the cauliflower a nice color. Spread the cauliflower mashed potatoes over the sautéed veggies in small casserole dishes, then sprinkle over with the finely chopped chives. Enjoy!

DECADENT CREAMY CHOCOLATE MOUSSE

Can we say "Hell, yeah!" to a guilt-free chocolate mousse? The raw cocoa and avocado are the perfect combination for a load of great fats. Rest assured your palate and digestive system will thank you for this one—not to mention it is super easy to make!

INGREDIENTS:

1 ripe avocado, pitted and scooped out of its skin

¼ cup maple syrup or agave nectar

¼ cup cocoa powder/raw cacao powder

¼ cup water

2 tsp vanilla extract

¼ tsp sea salt

DIRECTIONS:

Blend avocado, maple syrup or agave nectar, cocoa powder, vanilla extract and sea salt in a blender. Gradually add 1 Tablespoon of water at a time to achieve a creamy consistency.

Chill, then serve with a topping of shredded raw almonds. For extra sweetness, have with a topping of fresh organic raspberries and enjoy!

EACH ONE OF US HAS A UNIQUE PALETTE. SOME OF US LIKE IT SPICY, SWEETER, OR LIGHT–MILD.

ABOUT IBETLIZA

Ibetliza Frias is a lover of all things Holistic and promotes female empowerment through consistent Self-Care regimens. She began her own healing journey in her early twenties while on the pathway to self-awareness. She had a deep yearning for connection, contentment and acceptance. As an introvert, she did not necessarily feel she fit in and shied away from social settings, choosing to spend time alone.

Her entire mental dynamic shifted when a close friend invited her to a sister circle. A female gathering of this nature had been a foreign concept to her up until then. Sister Circles changed Ibetliza's life; they became a vehicle for self-love and connection. She began to uncover her authenticity and created a place of trust and sanctuary where she experienced deep healing of covered wounds. She said goodbye to negative emotional constructs like unworthiness, the need to hide and denying herself life's pleasures.

Relishing the new journey, she immersed herself in guiding books, soul regimens and creating an empowering tool chest, and now moves through life with energetic confidence and endless self-love.

Based on this soul stirring work, Ibetliza has cultivated a natural way of inspiring women. She is the founder of Divine Motherhood, a one-on-one health coaching practice and private chef service in New York and New Jersey. She is often found testing recipes and whipping up unforgettable dishes for her clients, and uses her life experiences to guide them towards an enriched and fulfilling path.

Ibetliza's mission is to convey the secrets to "having it all" through sacred self-care and having a spiritual relationship with Self. She is committed to passing on the gifts of self-awareness and a lighted path to more and better.

Visit Ibetliza at: http://www.divine-motherhood.com ✳

"

THE MORE YOU
LET GO OF THE
RULES AND MAKE
ROOM FOR FUN
AND PLAY, THE
MORE YOUR
CONFIDENCE BUILDS
AND YOU'RE GUIDED
BY YOUR OWN
CREATIVITY.

4

HEALING YOUR MONEY STORY

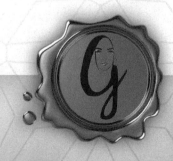

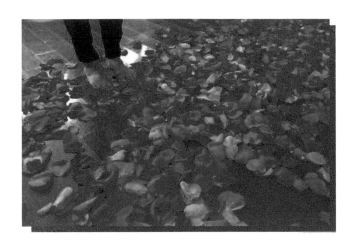

MONEY WAS A TOPIC I
AVOIDED LIKE THE SIGHT
OF CHOPPED LIVER. Just the
thought of it gave me intense knots in my belly.
In my household, I remember loud arguments
around money and financial struggles while my dad worked full time and
my mother was in school. As a child, I felt a lot of shame and tried my
best around my peers to pretend this wasn't happening. Conversations
of "we can't afford this" ran rampant as a child. As I transitioned into
adulthood, I felt embarrassed at the thought of sharing my deep fears
around this with close friends. Would they judge me? Was I was secretly
cursed when it came to money? I desperately wanted freedom around
these thoughts that were stirred up inside of me. The thing was I had
no idea where to begin. Managing money and creating wealth was not a
conversation that I knew any women were having.

　　As an adult this was what was running my life when it came to any
choice that needed to be made.

These limiting beliefs consumed what was supposed to be my precious waking moments. I was constantly anxious when going out to dinner with people, secretly praying they would pick up the tab. All of my dreams had been tabled into a "someday I will do that" file, like traveling the world or going out for a decadent meal. Truth be told, I had developed a secret fantasy of a Prince Charming whisking me off to five star restaurants and taking me on fancy trips! My scarcity thinking was rambling on in my head about ways I could live my dream life—and not have to pay for it on my own.

But as I was hanging out with these fierce goddesses who wanted me to live my best life, I knew eventually I would have to face my money story. I deeply desired a feeling of freedom around this. But how? It took a few months to move through the resistance and look at the way I viewed money with a new set of eyes. I had to come to terms with the idea that I wasn't a victim around this, or that my upbringing didn't have to keep me in my current self-imposed state of suffering.

DEALING WITH SPREADSHEETS IN THE BEGINNING WAS CERTAINLY NOT MY IDEA OF SEXY.

My first money coach, Saadi, helped me disconnect my internal money dialogue from my parents' conversations. They had their way of looking at money, that was their legacy, and I was learning some powerful-ass tools to create my own. I was guided to value my time— something I had never connected with money. O-M-Goddess! Not once had I realized that, what I did with my time, who I spent it with— giving all this precious life force energy away—*could affect my flow of abundance.*

"HELLO, THERE, I'M YOUR FINANCIAL WAKE UP CALL!"

Dealing with spreadsheets in the beginning was certainly not my idea of sexy. But we all know—what we resist persists. I was sick enough of being short on the rent, turning down invitations to travel to fabulous places with other goddesses, and feeling that money just wasn't meant to stay in MY bank account.

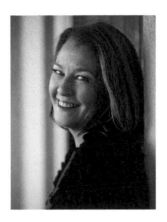

MAGGIE OSTARA

GODDESS MONEY TIP: I learned how to save and pay myself first. GODDESS CROWN ADJUSTED!

Learning to rely on having my own back when it came to finances was a new muscle I practiced daily—and eventually my outdated "Prince Charming" fantasy was issued a death sentence!

During my journey, I had the pleasure of working with Maggie Ostara. I knew my knowledge of transforming my relationship with money was far from over; it had honestly just begun! She arrived in my life at a time when I was ready to expand my business, yet I could feel sheer terror each time I thought of making a move.

When we began working together, I was only doing my one-day Goddess On The Go events. I had begun casually exploring luxurious destination retreats and was in the midst of creating my Royal Goddess Immersion Program in-person circles. Maggie's brilliant advice of "not waiting until everything is perfect to begin" was like gold melting onto my ears. In two months I had filled both my circle and retreat! Her priceless coaching to infuse breath work, self-care, and action supported all of this into reality. There was a new level of abundant flow and trust!

I finally felt as if I was in a healthy relationship with money. My dreams of traveling the world were happening, goddesses! Talk about wanting to pinch yourself some mornings 'cause you're so excited! Within a year and a half I traveled to Italy, Greece, Croatia, Bali, Hawaii, Bermuda, and Tulum, paying cash for each trip. This was all about so much more than a luxurious vacation—it was a journey of self-love that was preparing me for my divine mate.

When he did show up, it wasn't in the way I had imagined! My honey moved from Detroit to be with me at a time when I was soaring in every area of my life and he was beginning his all over again. My head tried to talk me out of it but my soul knew that this was the person I needed to be with.

When he arrived, he got the good ol' NYC ass kicking that 99% of people get when they move here! The jobs he received were underpaying him and it began to create tension between us. In the midst of all of this—I got pregnant.

Stress and anxiety triggered up my money stuff. Anxiety, too! For the first time, we were arguing about everything! It felt as if our relationship was being tested to see if we would throw the towel in on our love or learn how to grow from this. Somehow his constant jokes and him being an amazing dad to our daughter helped us make it through some of the darkest moments.

Through our two-year challenge in a new partnership, I had gotten back into $20,000 in credit card debt and went through a large chunk of savings. My sisters suggested taking Barbara Stanny's "One Year To Wealth" course, which was all about learning to invest. Growing up in scarcity, I thought only privileged white men had the scoop on that. Being at one of the lowest times in my life that I had ever been, I was scared to spend the money to sign up. Yet I could hear that little voice nudging me to do it. Eventually I gave in to my desire and registered, trusting that things would shift.

I PAID OFF ALL OF MY CREDIT CARD DEBT. INSERT DANCE PARTY!

Working with Barbara, my flow with money skyrocketed. I learned about things that had baffled the shit out of me in the past like stocks, real estate, bonds, and investing in my family's future. *Taking risks became FUN!* Like feeling confident to hire a certified financial planner to begin working together with me and my honey, having someone hold me accountable to be bold around my finances, and I paid off all of my credit card debt. Insert dance party!

Money is energy, and for many of us, there are plenty of deep-seated emotions tied to it that feel very real. Goddesses, here is where you may want to crawl under a rock and hide. I want to gently say, **"Do not SKIP this chapter and the inner work that each one of these bad ass money guidesses has created for you."** We often wonder why the second chakra represents both money and intimacy. They are more connected than Donald Trump to the color orange! If you desire a healthy affinity with romantic love you must throw on your most fabulous Agent Provocateur and get ready to develop a steaming-hot rendezvous with . . . money! ✳

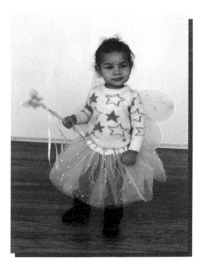

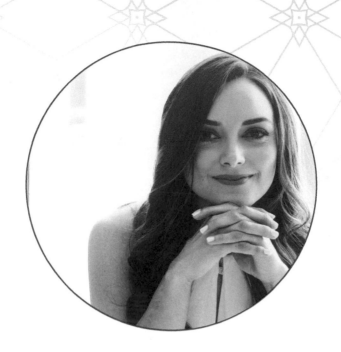

Money

MONEY MOJO

Divinely Contributed by

BRITTNEY CASTRO

Introduction

MANY OF US TOSS OUR MONTHLY BANK STATEMENTS IN THE "DO NOT OPEN" PILE, dreading to look at overdraft charges or how much we may have spent on fancy lattes. To my *avoiders*—this is a death sentence to our flow of abundance. We actually, as women, need to be in the know of what's going on in *all* areas of our lives. In our society, there's still an outdated mentality that men make and manage all the money. I give the middle finger to that dinosaur way of thinking, and so does my dear friend Brittney Castro. After developing her own empowering relationship with her finances, this goddess knew it was her mission to free up other women from their woes!

Don't assume I'm talking about some stuffy financial planner here, goddesses! Brittney's work is all about bringing in the feminine energy and fun, balancing that out with some realness and practical tools so you get to upgrade your money reality. She knows the importance of altering your fear so you can joyride with your dollars instead.

One of the brilliant tools she created is called the "money date"—I do this every Saturday morning! To set the tone, pour yourself a glass of Pellegrino, have a plate of your desired treats waiting for you, and throw on some feel good mellow music in the background. This is a sacred time for you and your finances.

Now, go woo yourself into a money making badass! ✳

"

WHEN YOU
LOVE YOUR MONEY,
YOUR MONEY WILL
LOVE YOU BACK.
AND THAT
MUTUAL LOVE
WILL MAKE
YOU RICH.

GENERALLY SPEAKING,
MEN DON'T HAVE THESE SAME
ROADBLOCKS OF ASKING FOR
MONEY, AS THEY ARE NATURAL
PIONEERS AND HAVE VERY LITTLE
ATTACHMENT TO QUESTIONING
THEIR VALUE.

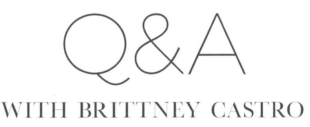

WITH BRITTNEY CASTRO

L: **What do you see as the most replayed story women carry when it comes to their money?**

B: The most common fear I've noticed is that women carry a story that says they will never be able to figure their financial situation out. There's a large "old" conditioning of judgment where we often tell ourselves we "should have this together by now." This stops us from asking important questions and even has us avoid looking at our money.

L: **Do you think we carry an internal guilt in our lineage as women about earning too much cash?**

B: Yes. Historically thinking, women have been more of the gatherers, nurturers, and lovers. Once we go into the work force, that question of self-worth comes up. We question whether we are good enough to accept large amounts of money for our time or services. We doubt whether we have enough experience, or worry that we may be a fraud. Generally speaking, men don't have these same roadblocks of asking for money, as they are natural pioneers and have very little attachment to questioning their value.

L: **If I could put you on loudspeaker right now what would you want every woman to know?**

B: If one woman can do it, so can you. Women who have achieved financial success and taken control over their money don't have anything different inside of them than you. Learn to engage with your own money in a loving, positive and conscious way. Then make a choice to commit to looking at your money and relating to your money from an empowered point of view.

WHEN YOU SHOW YOUR MONEY
LOVE BY TAKING CARE OF IT AND
MANAGING IT PROPERLY,
YOU CONTINUE TO CREATE THE
SPACE TO ALLOW FOR MORE MONEY
TO COME INTO YOUR LIFE.

Money Ritual: Weekly Money Date!

One of the best ways to show your money the love it deserves is by having a weekly date with it. Commit to a weekly "Money Date"—an hour a week that you devote to things like reviewing your accounts, updating your budget and tracking your progress towards financial goals. A weekly date keeps your money management tasks bite-sized so they never become so big that you dread doing them.

The weekly check-in also allows you to be more flexible with your money week after week, which then allows you to be more likely to stay on track with your budget and financial goals. For example, if you overspend one week eating out, then you can re-adjust the next week by saving in another area. By having weekly money dates, you simply are able to stay more conscious and present with your money and spending behaviors. This helps free up your mind the rest of the week, so you're not always thinking and worrying about your money.

Steps for Setting up a Weekly Money Date:

1. **SET UP A RECURRING EVENT IN YOUR CALENDAR FOR A WEEKLY MONEY DATE:** Choose a day and time that you can realistically commit to a weekly one hour date with your money. Once you select the day and time, set up a recurring event in your calendar to help you stay accountable toward getting it down. If it's in your calendar every week, you're more likely to get it done—and not put it off like most people do.

2. **WHAT TO DO DURING YOUR MONEY DATE:** During your Money Date, you should update your budget, review any upcoming expenses, pay bills (although you should automate those as much as possible), review your accounts for accuracy and handle any other pressing financial matters. You can also use this time to learn about a new financial topic and read a finance blog or finance article to help you expand your financial wisdom.

3. MAKE YOUR MONEY DATES AS FUN AS POSSIBLE: To help you stay committed to weekly Money Dates, make them as fun as you possibly can for yourself. Listen to music, dance, light candles or do anything else that makes the personal finance process fun for you. You can even reward yourself with a glass of wine once you complete your Money Date. The more fun you have with your Money Dates, the more likely it is that you'll continue to do it—and consistency is what counts.

4. BRING POSITIVE, LOVING ENERGY INTO YOUR MONEY DATES: Finally, always check in with yourself right before you have your Money Dates to ensure your feelings are full of love, peace, joy and bliss. So often, women are not aware of their feelings when dealing with money, and enter into their money relationship in a state of fear, stress, confusion, and overwhelm. Remember, you are the driver of your financial life and get to choose how you feel about your money, so make sure you check any negativity at the door and shift into the right mindset when you begin your money date.

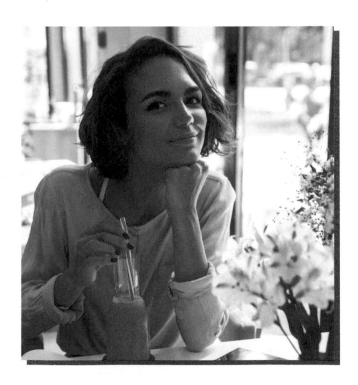

When you show your money love by taking care of it and managing it properly, you continue to create the space to allow for more money to come into your life. **The bottom line: When you love your money, your money will love you back. And that mutual love will make you rich.**

MONEY RITUAL: WEEKLY MONEY DATE!

Brittney Castro, CFP®, AAMS®, CRPC® is the founder and CEO of Financially Wise Women, a Los Angeles-based financial planning firm whose mission is to teach women and couples the art of managing their money the fun and simple way. As a Certified Financial Planner™, Chartered Retirement Planning Counselor, Accredited Asset Management Specialist, entrepreneur and speaker, Brittney works with busy professional women and couples who are ready to make their finances work for them and use their money to live the lives of their dreams. After years of working in the male-dominated world of financial planning, Brittney realized she wanted to work with clients the same way she talks about money with her girlfriends–in a smart, personal, feminine way that's compassionate, fun and nonjudgmental.

Brittney has become a well-known financial expert and a go-to resource for national media outlets. She's been featured on CNN, CNBC, The Wall Street Journal, The New York Times, CBS, KTLA, Fox 11 News, Glamour, Elle, Marie Claire, Darling, Entrepreneur, Woman's World, Financial Planning, Investment News, Registered Rep magazine and many more. She's also a coveted speaker and host, and she loves spreading her wisdom about finance, entrepreneurship and smart investing to the masses.

For more information, visit: www.financiallywisewomen.com or follow her on social media @BrittneyCastro ✳

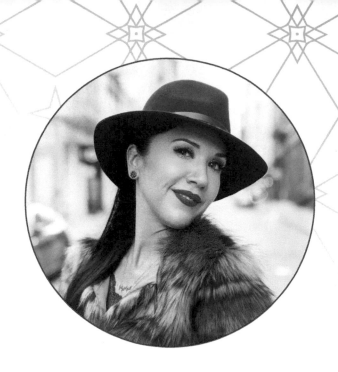

Money

THE
FEMMEPRENEUR
WITHIN

✳

Divinely Contributed by

INGRID ARNA

Introduction

THERE'S SOMETHING THAT INTERNALLY SHIFTS WHEN A WOMAN IS REFLECTED BACK the best parts of herself that she has forgotten. During our first Skype call five years ago, I could feel Ingrid mirror back to me my own worth. I was in a challenging business partnership that was affecting my confidence and the way I valued what I was bringing to the table. She helped me to release whatever thoughts were in the way and BOOM the next thing you know I ended that alliance and doubled my rates.

Ingrid guides you to shake up your outdated value system so you can begin respecting the life force energy that you bring into your businesses. Goddesses, stop shrinking when it comes to setting your prices and owning your value. Throw on your sparkly ball gowns and rock that sales call out!

Ingrid, like myself, knows that our time on this planet is precious. We can no longer live mediocre lives, chase scarcity, or put up with "just enough." Ingrid reminds us that the money will come when we love the shizz out of ourselves and focus on being deep in service to others. When women own their inherent power, we will change the world. ✳

"

SUCCESS IS NOT
JUST LOVING
WHAT YOU DO BUT
HOW YOU DO IT.
IF YOU WANT TO
MAKE AN IMPACT,
YOU NEED TO
MAKE MONEY
TO DO IT.

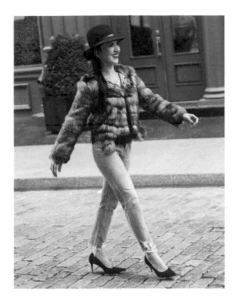

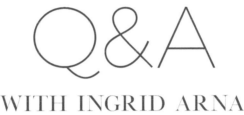

WITH INGRID ARNA

L: Why do so many women suffer from the undercharging disease and then take it even further by overcompensating for their services?

I: I honestly believe this starts from a deep desire to serve but also includes a desire to be kind and be liked, which in many ways is such a beautiful gift to the world. But what tends to happen is so many women then stay trapped in struggle. It all starts from an early age when we are often told that being strong or asking for "more" is selfish instead of self-FULL.

At the end of the day, to really be empowered and serve at a deeper level, financial struggle—which always becomes an emotional and physical struggle—needs to be cured. The overcompensation stems from the same disease to please and leads to overwork and depletion. The truth is that, if you want to heal your bank account, you have to heal your need to be liked and step into being great.

Serving at our highest means we need to be paid well to make the impact we desire to make. The world really needs women to rise because we genuinely care. But we have to begin to do this from a position of financial empowerment and ditch the shame. Money is a wonderful healing tool when used for good. I think women need to get this into their bones! When you love yourself, you create a new reality with money. You also learn to master the law of energy, including how to set boundaries and how to sell and rock your business like a CEO Diva.

THE TRUTH IS THAT, IF YOU WANT TO HEAL YOUR BANK ACCOUNT, YOU HAVE TO HEAL YOUR NEED TO BE LIKED AND STEP INTO BEING GREAT.

L: **So many women find it difficult setting healthy boundaries. Can you explain how we got here and how to break the cycle?**

I: I think once again this is conditioning that begins from a young age. We are taught to be pretty and popular, and we get GOLD stars when we score these achievements.

We're not often told to stand out, shake up the status quo, say it like it is, or be strong. So in order to please and get the love and approval that we are also conditioned to seek, we naturally have really flimsy boundaries. Some women have none at all. It's not easy to break the pattern, but it is absolutely doable!

WE NEED MORE SISTERS TO RISE INTO POWER TO CREATE THE SHIFTS WE NEED GLOBALLY. AS EACH WOMAN RISES, WE LIGHT A FLAME IN ANOTHER.

The truth is MONEY IS INNOCENT! We just project all our beliefs, and all those beliefs we've taken on from others about money, *onto* money, which leads to a lot of dysfunction, struggle and fear. "Oh, poor money!" You have to laugh at that sentence!

To release any residual ill will we have towards money, we must feel into our perceptions and beliefs about it and, in doing so, clearly see the cause of our diseased relationship with money. I truly believe that a shift in perception and a willingness to get to the bottom of why we block money, over spend, under charge, feel guilty when receiving money or ashamed for not having enough, feel scared around it, and still feel unsafe and needy despite making great money, is exactly the sacred step we need to take to set ourselves free from money struggles forever. And this is exactly what I walk you through in **Money Rituals 1 & 2** below.

L: **You talk so much about unconscious incompetence and how it relates to women building their financial success. Can you share more about this, as well as any tools for financial wellbeing?**

I: The biggest challenge I see consistently for my clients is a lack of belief in their own brilliance. What follows is an inability to grow a sustainable business and a nourishing life. In order for a woman to serve and rise financially, she needs to build it from within. Otherwise, she can feel like she's drowning in six figures!

With love and advanced strategy, I guide my clients to create financially lucrative and soul-aligned businesses. With over 20 years of experience in business, I know what works and what doesn't. Unless you build a company with a solid foundation, with systems that allow you to grow into seven figures, you run the risk of driving yourself and your relationships into the ground.

My work is about ensuring that women not only make great money but that they create businesses that give them true FREEDOM. Success is not just loving what you do but how you do it. If you want to make an impact, you need to make money to do it. In short, I activate femmepreneurs to own their brilliance and charge what they are worth so they can make the impact they were born to make!

I love nothing more than seeing other women step into their power to create lucrative brands that not only change their own lives but change the world. The Dalai Lama said, "The Western woman will change the world."

I fully agree with this statement; in fact, we are already doing it. On the flip side, I also see a lot of struggle. We need more sisters to rise into power to create the shifts we need globally. As each woman rises, we light a flame in another. Women are born leaders. We just have to follow our vision and courage.

Money Ritual #1

Breaking Negative Patterns

In order to heal your money karma drama, you need to begin to release the false beliefs about money and your worth. Here is a simple yet powerful ritual for you to begin the process: Writing down the five ways you feel disrespected, drained or overwhelmed.

Once you have identified the five areas of your life that you feel exhaust you, you can then ask, "How can I change that? If I was in my highest power and truly loved myself, how would I set up new boundaries in my business, personal life, or with my children?" And next I would ask myself what I need to a) stop doing, b) heal, or c) release that perpetuates this cycle.

Doing an exercise like this is extremely powerful and life changing. Awareness is key to becoming the CEO DIVA of your own life. Each day we have the opportunity to change the course of our lives with every thought, feeling and action. It's really quite amazing!

As you take a moment to tune inwards, please list all the money beliefs you have that are causing you pain. Put your hand on your heart and say: *Darling LOVE, what do you need for me to release? What is now stopping me from receiving financial flow and divine abundance?*

Examples of beliefs that may be holding you back from receiving divine compensation:

- I don't deserve money.
- Money causes pain and manipulation.
- I'm a greedy bitch to want money.
- Who am I to charge that much?
- If I am a good woman and want to help others, I can't make great money or build a business.
- I have to bleed or sacrifice myself in some way to receive money.
- Money isn't spiritual.
- I don't need money.
- Money isn't important.
- I am a bad person and too materialistic to want money.
- I should be punished if I am to make a lot of money.

SUCCESS IS NOT JUST LOVING WHAT YOU DO BUT HOW YOU DO IT.

Money Ritual #2

The Rich CEO Diva Goddess Life Mantra

The money will come when you own your inherent power and stop waiting for money to give you power or to prove your worth.

It's simply a form of energy; it doesn't prove your value or your worth.

When money shows up in your life, it proves that you've attached an energy exchange (a financial one—there are many) to your work or service and that you desire the pleasure and choice that comes when you have financial freedom.

Don't be fooled, though. Financial freedom comes when you realize that you're always free to receive money. You're always free to desire it. You are always free to give your work a monetary value that makes you feel really good. But we all know that you and your work are limitless, and that, too, is energy. It's all energy. It's all belief. It's all about our values and our relationship to our creative power. Chant this mantra with deep feeling and trust:

(Download the FREE guided audio here: http://ceodiva.com/ meditation/)

Dear Creator of all that is,
Please allow me to release all emotions that are not love with ease and grace. Shift me into a woman who knows without a shadow of a doubt that I deserve ease, flow, radiance, abundance, fun, love, rest and pleasure in my life. I now release all struggle and force.

My business is now surrounded by DIVINE light and builds with GRACE.

I have wonderful new clients, partners and mentors who truly support me and my vision, but most of all I support myself. I trust and believe in my ability to serve others and to make great money doing what I do. My life is full of heart-centered, divine and soulful relationships. My clients are incredible, soulful women (or men) who totally align with my teachings.

I take the time needed to slow down and to put myself, my health and my loved ones first. I am now building the most supportive team, which allows me to do more of what I love in the business. I do not need to work alone as I magnetically attract a posse of co-creative alliances and partnerships into my life and business.

I communicate with strength and love. I clearly own my voice and express myself with passion and poise. I am healthy, radiant and divine. My body is rich with beauty and radiance. My energy is consistent and strong. I am in tune with my emotions and my intuition. I feel incredible.

I totally trust myself and my new rich life, which is full of love, flow and divine abundance.

I am at PEACE.

I am POWERFUL.

I am LOVE.

I am a RICH CEO DIVA GODDESS in every cell of my being.

I speak with LOVE, CLARITY and POWER about my business offerings.

I honor money, I honor my work and I honor myself, and in doing so I inspire others to step into *their* Divine power.

I do not chase clients. They come to me with ease. I am so rich, full and in love with the service I provide that all desperation, lack or need to make this happen is replaced with a sense of humble, calm confidence and faith. I may not know the exact path, but I do see clearly into my future. That is all I need. I now focus purely on how I want to feel and that is the magnetic power that allows me to attract abundance with Divine ease. I listen to my soul. I connect with the Divine, and I move through life with a deep sense of TRUST and JOY.

As I move from fear into LOVE, financial miracles flow into my life with Divine Grace.

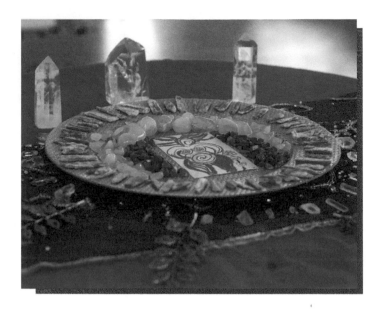

ABOUT INGRID

Ingrid Arna is a leading Intuitive Business Strategist and the founder of CEO Diva Business School and the Gucci of online business programs, High-End Empire. She's been endorsed by Kate Winslet for her work and has been featured in Cosmopolitan, InStyle, Huffington Post, Good Health Magazine and on The Steve Harvey Show. Ingrid leads visionary entrepreneurs into conscious wealth and global impact without sacrificing their souls. The only New Year's resolutions she's been able to stick to since becoming a mother is quadrupling her prices and giving up her thongs for granny pants. She's never been happier.

If you want to get your hands on Ingrid's FREE video program to shift how you make money forever, sign up at: http://www.ingridarna.com/smm

In this FREE training program, you'll shift from charging peanuts to selling high-end programs like a diva who owns her magic. Discover how Ingrid went from struggling to sell $150 sessions to selling $30k packages with GRACE and INTEGRITY.

Visit Ingrid at: www.ingridarna.com ✳

"

WE NEED MORE
SISTERS TO RISE
INTO POWER TO
CREATE THE SHIFTS
WE NEED GLOBALLY.
AS EACH WOMAN
RISES, WE LIGHT
A FLAME IN
ANOTHER.

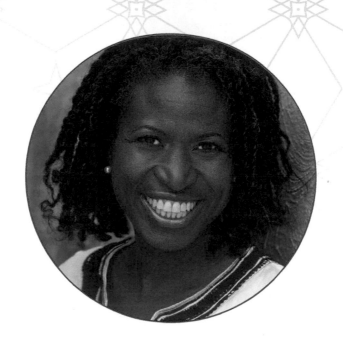

Money

—————

BURIED
TREASURE

✳

Divinely Contributed by

KARLA LIGHTFOOT

Introduction

WHEN I BOOKED MY FIRST SESSION WITH KARLA, I WAS AT A CROSSROADS AROUND love. I was in a turbulent state of "hot mess." I found myself spending hours obsessing about a certain someone, which was taking away precious hours from my business. My ebb and flow of money was totally "stuck." Karla got right down to the nitty gritty of it and steered me to seeing that I was carrying around a story of *not deserving* and *not enough*. Ugghhh—again?! We worked on healing this layer of emotions so I could steer clear of the love drama and step deeper into my divine purpose. I could feel it was time to release this lover and, instead of being pissed off, I ended the relationship in appreciation. Keeping my space clear and open, abundance began to gush back in. The next thing I remember I experienced an opening to my dollars flowing.

Karla's own story of clearing her limiting beliefs around abundance through her hypnosis practice is SO juicy!

(And on a delicious side note, if it was not for Karla's magical hypno-birthing skills, I would never have had the patience to be present for the 6 hours and 11 minutes it took for my daughter Cariel to come out of that birth canal!) ✳

"

IN HYPNOTHERAPY, WE WORK WITH THE SUBCONSCIOUS TO PROCESS THE OLD, RETRAIN YOUR BRAIN AND BODY, AND REINFORCE THE NEW!

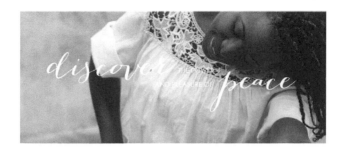

Q&A

WITH KARLA LIGHTFOOT

L: **Karla, let's start off with a little bit about what hypnosis is and what it is not. Many people may feel it's too "woo-woo." For me, personally, it was life-altering—especially the experience my partner and I had in the delivery room!**

K: Hypnosis is NOT mind control. In fact, hypnosis frees the mind and the body! Hypnosis is simply a highly relaxed state in which your mind remains focused and open to positive suggestion. In this natural state, it's easier to work with the mind to change the habits, thoughts, beliefs, and ideas that no longer serve or support you. The sensation can be similar to yoga, savasana, meditation, acupuncture, massage or anything else that's pleasurable and relaxing. However, with hypnosis, there is a specific focus.

Many have had hypnosis experiences or memories that involve stage hypnosis, or yes, even cartoons. With stage hypnosis, the specific focus may be to let go and have a good time, so you'll see people quacking like ducks or doing other seemingly "crazy" things. It's important to remember that the brain's main objective is to keep you safe and comfortable, to help you survive, and that you cannot—and will not—do anything against your will while in hypnosis. While you are open to the suggestion of imagining or doing certain things, you are conscious and completely aware of your actions at all times. You cannot get stuck in hypnosis either, and, similar to sleep, you can come up and out of a hypnotic state by choosing to do so at anytime.

In hypnotherapy, we work with the subconscious to process the old, retrain your brain and body, and reinforce the new!

. . . I HAD EMBODIED THE IDEA THAT I WAS A 'FINANCIAL BURDEN' AND CARRIED OUT THE NECESSARY HABITS TO PROVE IT.

L: **I know I totally piqued the goddesses' desire to hear your own story around money. Would you be so generous as to share more about that?**

K: Growing up, my parents were very generous in terms of schooling, camp, amazing travel experiences and the like. Many would agree that I have cool parents who provided me with a great childhood. I have always been very appreciative, but after college I noticed I was starting to feel guilty. So guilty that, as I grew older, I started to feel like a financial burden. I thought they could have been doing better things with all that money.

Although I felt guilty, I began to rack up debt and get myself in situations where I needed to borrow money *pronto* in order to maintain my credit or be "okay." This is what we tend to do when we have certain beliefs—we either live the beliefs out or we do our best to prove that the opposite is true. (For instance, we may become a complete "burden" or hyper-independent to the extent that we cannot and will not allow or accept help from others.)

Well, I had embodied the idea that I was a "financial burden" and carried out the necessary habits to prove it. And to be clear, as always, there were a ton of other beliefs layered in there—I believed I wasn't worthy of making or receiving a lot of money, money was bad, that there wasn't enough to go around, people who made a lot of money were troubled or unkind, money causes problems, it was wrong to make or desire to make more money when you had enough. Phew—the list goes on!

With hypnotherapy, I gained clarity around my money beliefs and patterns, and with support, I began shifting the habits and patterns so I could create a healthy relationship with money. To this day, I pay attention to that relationship. I use affirmations and take action steps that support me in my money journey and reinforce any new, more supportive ways of thinking and being.

L: **How long does it take for people to start seeing the potent effects of the hypnotherapy session after working with you?**

K: People experience clear effects as soon as a session or two. Often, I suggest 6-9 sessions to fully support the person and the process.

Money Ritual: "Dear Universe . . ."

I believe that everyone is capable of co-creating change and healing themselves. Like anything, hypnosis is a practice. When you work with a compassionate witness or co-pilot, like a hypnotherapist or coach, it can move things along a lot faster. Others can see the limiting thoughts, beliefs and behaviors that you are unable to see for yourself.

Here's a great exercise I prescribe and use for transforming financial issues and increasing the flow of money into your life:

1. WRITE A "MAD LETTER" ABOUT MONEY, TO MONEY, TO YOURSELF, OR ANY OTHERS INVOLVED, THE UNIVERSE, YOUR HIGHER SELF, GOD. Is there something about moola that makes you angry, upset, frustrated, annoyed? Do you think you decided something about money, or learned something from your parents or relatives, or from society? Did something "bad" happen to or around you with regard to money? Did someone else always give you money so you never had to think about it?

WHEN YOU FEEL LIKE YOU'VE GOTTEN IT ALL OUT, SIMPLY BURN IT! IN A SAFE PLACE, OF COURSE.

These questions are meant to take you on your own journey of money discovery and dismantle the ideas that no longer serve you. Each of us has unique money and Life experiences. Spend some time to uncover yours. Talk it out, go down memory lane, write it down, notice how it feels in your body and where you feel it. Keep sharing your frustrations or confusion on paper—make it a physical act—let the tears flow, breathe deeply, stomp your feet or howl if you need to! When you feel like you've gotten it all out, simply burn it! In a safe place, of course. A metal sink, an ashtray or a pot that can be covered. Watch it burn and drift away into nothingness. You might even repeat, "Yes, I'm done with that," out loud or do a celebration dance.

All thoughts and beliefs come from what we make up and/or decide about our experience. So we can always feel free to change our minds and actions when our old decisions no longer serve us. Thoughts, beliefs, ideas, and money itself are all energy. Every "thing" is energy—and beliefs, just like energy, have the ability to be neutral, to shift and transform as quickly and easily as they are formed.

Let them.

2. NOW WRITE A LETTER THAT DETAILS YOUR NEW RELATIONSHIP WITH MONEY, WHAT YOU WOULD RATHER EXPERIENCE. Write each statement in the present tense and focus on the positive—what you desire more of. You'll notice that the letter becomes one giant affirmation.

You might start with something like, "I am so grateful money and I are (becoming) friends now. Because I have a healthier relationship with money now, I have more money in my life. I take better care of myself and my family, and that feels good. Great ideas, new clients, and payments come to me easily. I now enjoy a surplus cash flow. I receive money from expected and unexpected places. I am living in the flow."

Continue writing in the present. As if *the Now* is already here and unfolding.

Don't burn this one. In fact, read, write or repeat your statement aloud every day, morning and night, for the next 90 days or more.

3. VISUALIZE AND ACTUALIZE. Use the faculties of your subconscious mind to imagine, sense, feel and see the money, the clients, and all of the abundance around you, 2-3 times daily or more. You can close your eyes wherever you are, take 3 deep, slow breaths, and allow yourself to imagine the examples below or any of your own financial abundance imagery. You can imagine, sense,

feel, or think about a giant net—whisking it through the sky or the ocean and filling it up with all the stars or ocean treasures you desire. You can imagine money raining or pouring down on you, see your appointment book filled for months in advance, or even online payments being deposited into your bank account. Or again, any other imagery that supports you in prospering. You might also imagine any obstacles and see yourself taking the action you need to move through them. You'll also take inspired baby action steps toward your financial desires daily. Let it be easy and fun!

SINCE YOUR SUBCONSCIOUS MIND IS BUILT TO CARRY OUT ORDERS FOR YOU, IT CAN BEGIN TO SUPPORT YOU IN ESTABLISHING AND MAINTAINING THIS NEW RELATIONSHIP WITH MONEY.

4. **A RITUAL FOR CHANGE.** You're learning to work with your mind, identifying and letting go of the ideas and beliefs that no longer support you. You are guiding your mind to focus on the Now and how you wish to live. Since your subconscious doesn't know fact from fiction, and is built to carry out orders and keep you safe, with this newfound clarity, it can begin to support you in establishing and maintaining your new relationship with money. To bolster it all, you're reading your letter, using imagery, and your emotions daily to co-create in the now, and build a new connection with money and prosperity.

    Hypnosis is a practice, just like meditation or prayer or yoga. It's important to pay attention and continually reinforce the new. Whether you find yourself feeling extraordinary resistance, or whether you move through the exercise with ease: practice, practice, practice. *The same way you repeated the old patterns is the same way you create the new ones . . . affirmation and repetition.*

Keep working the steps until your experience feels lighter and more natural. You can always seek out support to move you along more easily. Your mind and body are your most powerful assets. With consistent awareness, intention and action, you can un-learn absolutely anything and co-create the life you desire!

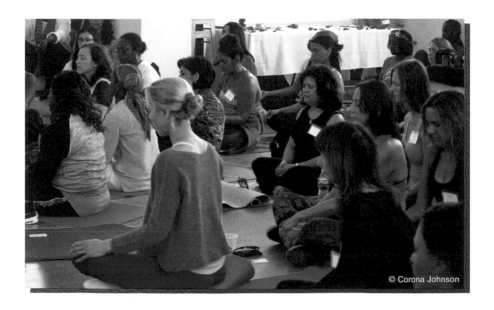
© Corona Johnson

ABOUT KARLA

Karla is a clinical hypnotherapist and life explorer who teaches people to harness the power of the subconscious to transform their lives— physically, emotionally, mentally, energetically and spiritually. She has worked with thousands, including stay-at-home moms, entrepreneurs, and professionals, to dissolve the limiting beliefs, fears, and behaviors that prevent us from living out our dreams.

Karla has used self-hypnosis to meet and marry her life partner and soulmate, dial down physical pain (she stuck a needle through her hand without feeling pain!), and dissolve the fear of public speaking, to name a few. She is a graduate of Wellesley College, the Columbia Graduate School of Journalism and the Hypnotherapy Academy of America in New Mexico. Her favorite pastime is to be in the Now, enjoying life— breathing, laughing, dancing, and having fun.

Many tell her she lights up a room, a subway, the city...with her positive energy. Most of all, she is committed to helping others to declutter their minds and SHINE. She believes that, with the right mind and heart, absolutely anything is possible!

Visit Karla at: www.karlalightfoot.com ✳

"

HYPNOSIS IS A
PRACTICE,
JUST LIKE
MEDITATION OR
PRAYER OR YOGA.
IT'S IMPORTANT
TO PAY ATTENTION
AND CONTINUALLY
REINFORCE
THE NEW.

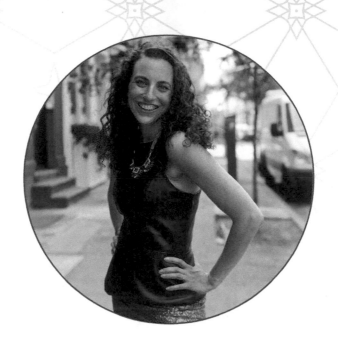

Money

EXPANDING
UNIVERSE

✳

Divinely Contributed by

JEN MAZER

Introduction

WHEN YOU'RE IN THE MIDDLE OF WRITING YOUR BOOK AND JUST SO HAPPEN TO MEET a fellow mama goddess who people call the "Queen Of Manifestation," you know she has to be a part of it! Jen and I met when I was five months pregnant, at a time when I wasn't feeling hopeful around motherhood or money. In about 30 minutes, Jen had snapped me out of my funk! Jen gave me a juicy peek into her life—from manifesting an unbelievable NYC apartment with a hot tub (where she lived rent-free for 10 years!) to helping clients manifest their first $60,000 months. In the past, Jen has randomly connected with top spiritual experts who have invited her to come speak on stage. She's not only the author of *Manifesting Made Easy*, she's also the cofounder of a game—*Sparked*. Jen is the bomb and the TRUUUTH!

As we all know, ABUN-DANCE isn't always about dollar signs. Sometimes it's about those things we magnetize towards us from vibrating so fucking high! You feel it when you receive an unexpected luxurious gift, or see an email pop in your inbox that makes you want to orgasm with delight, or when you're so dazzled by your own self that you meet your boo the moment you walk out the door with no makeup on!

I know you are ready for Jen to allure us with some of her MANIFESTING juju below. ✳

"

MANIFESTING
IS A LOT MORE
ABOUT ALLOWING
IN WHAT'S ALREADY
THERE FOR YOU,
VERSUS PUSHING
AND HUSTLING
TO MAKE THINGS
HAPPEN.

MANIFESTATION MEANS THAT,
THROUGH THE LAW OF ATTRACTION,
YOU CONSCIOUSLY CO-CREATE WITH
THE UNIVERSE TO EXPERIENCE
WHAT YOU DESIRE.

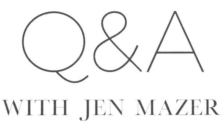

WITH JEN MAZER

L: **What does MANIFESTATION mean to you? In what ways can someone upgrade their skills and belief?**

J: Manifestation means that, through the law of attraction, you consciously co-create with the universe to experience what you desire. The first step in manifesting is to get clear on what you truly want so that the universe knows what to bring to you. We live in a reflective universe. So think of it like placing an order at a restaurant. If you don't know what you want to eat, the chefs in the kitchen can't make it for you. Set your intention by seeing it first, and you'll actually call it in. If you want to upgrade your manifesting skills, you can be grateful for your dreams in advance. Gratitude expands. First, make sure you're already keeping a gratitude journal and writing down what you're grateful for on a daily basis. This helps you view your entire life from the lens of gratitude. You'll notice that you start to look for evidence of things that make you grateful. Then start adding in gratitude statements for things that haven't yet shown up physically. It's another way of setting intentions that is much more powerful than affirmations alone. I go into all of the exact steps for manifesting in my book, *Manifesting Made Easy: How to Harness the Law of Attraction to Get What You Really Want!*

IMAGINATION IS ACTUALLY A FORM OF INTUITION.

L: **Why is it so difficult for many of us to call in the things we constantly find ourselves daydreaming about?**

J: People have difficulty manifesting what they really want because they lack the belief in themselves. You might say you want it—but somewhere deep down inside, you have limiting beliefs telling you why you can't have it. Start by realizing that manifesting is a lot more about allowing in what's already there for you, versus pushing and hustling to make things happen.

The fact that you have the idea or vision for something in the first place means that your dream is meant for you. Imagination is actually a form of intuition. So when you have a desire, know that it's coming from the universe as a gift. You're intuiting what's already on its way to you. Most people stop their manifestations right there at the idea stage. They don't believe their dreams are possible. An idea comes, and they instantly say, "No, it's too outrageous, will be too difficult, will take too much time, or is just plain crazy." So they don't take action on their dreams. They don't believe in their own power.

But what would happen if you had a vision and realized you're intuiting, not just dreaming? You'd have the missing piece of the manifestation puzzle: expectation. If you expect your dream to happen, you keep going until you reap the rewards. It's a bit like planting a seed and harvesting a vegetable. Once you plant the seed, you don't doubt that the vegetable will grow. You simply need to water it, and nurture it. The seed already has the knowledge within it to become that particular vegetable—just like you have everything within you that you need to live out your dreams. So trust in your visions, and have faith in the process. Expect everything to work out in your favor. You're way more supported than you know. You're already manifesting, whether you realize it or not.

L: **Can you share your most OUTRAGEOUS MANIFESTATION story?**

J: I manifested living rent-free in the East Village of Manhattan for 10 years in my own apartment with a Jacuzzi. It was my choice to leave the building. And when I did, I made over $76,000.

I had been living on the block and was drawn to this magical purple building. One day I started talking to a woman who was outside sweeping, and discovered she was living there rent-free. I was curious. She said there was a theater on the first floor where they put on concerts and plays. And she invited me to a play. I went with the intention of getting an apartment in the building. After the show, I talked with the people in charge, and simply asked if they had an apartment available. To my surprise, they said, "Yes. But only for someone who could make a website for the theater." I was in art school at NYU at the time and had never made a website before. But I was taking a computer class, and I knew I could make one. So I said yes. And the rest is history.

It was even more magical than I had imagined. Every Christmas, the great jazz musician Wynton Marsalis would come perform at our theater for us. And one year we recorded the concert and put out a live album that ended up being nominated for a Grammy! "Acting as if" and taking action before you're ready are two powerful lessons from my experience.

Money Ritual: "Raise Your Money Vibes Exercise"

You attract things to you that are a vibrational match to that which you're giving out. So in order to manifest more money, you'll want to raise your vibration to match the state of abundance you're calling in.

Answer the questions below in your journal or on a piece of paper, and you'll be well on your way to increasing your money vibes:

• What does abundance feel like to you?

• How do you want to feel when you have all of the money you desire?

Awesome! You don't actually need to have more money in order to feel abundant NOW. In fact, if you can do something to achieve the feeling now, then you'll magnetize the physical desire. And that will result in more of that feeling.

For example, if you want to feel free, what else can you do to feel free? Or if you want to feel secure, what else can you do to feel secure? Make sense?

• What can I do now to feel that way?

If abundance feels like freedom to you, maybe you drive your car with your windows down and blast music. Or you take a pole dancing class. *What would be fun for you to do TODAY to feel the way you want to feel?*

THEN TAKE ACTION!

You don't have to spend money to do this exercise. You can simply hang out in another part of town where you imagine yourself to be living. You could go to a car dealership and test drive a convertible to see how it feels to drive it around.

Even though you might not fully believe it yet on the inside, your outward behavior helps get you there. Think about it: Haven't you ever gotten a new haircut or a new outfit, and then you found yourself acting different? You were probably more confident afterwards, right?

So get dressed up, go out and have some fun!

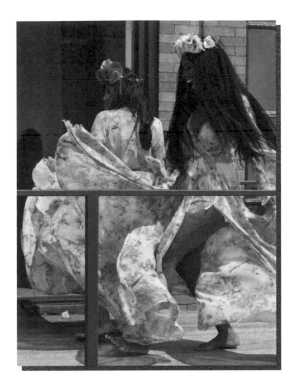

ABOUT JEN

Jen Mazer is the Queen of Manifestation. She's always been able to dream up outrageous adventures and actually live them out—from rubbing elbows at a small private cocktail party hosted by Martin Scorsese, to living rent-free in the East Village of Manhattan for 10 years, to paying off over $38,000 of debt in less than a year, having her artwork published in the New York Times, traveling the world, meeting the man of her dreams (a successful rock star), giving birth at home to a beautiful daughter, and starting a green school in Africa.

Jen is a sought-after transformational speaker and coach. She teaches people how to manifest their biggest dreams while making an impact on the world. She is known for her signature Manifestation Masters Program and Private Success Coaching.

Jen is also the cofounder of the new board game for women, "Sparked," available now. She has interviewed some of the world's biggest thought leaders through her series "Manifesting with the Masters."

Visit Jen at: www.queenofmanifestation.com ✳

5

FULL
SPECTRUM
BEAUTY

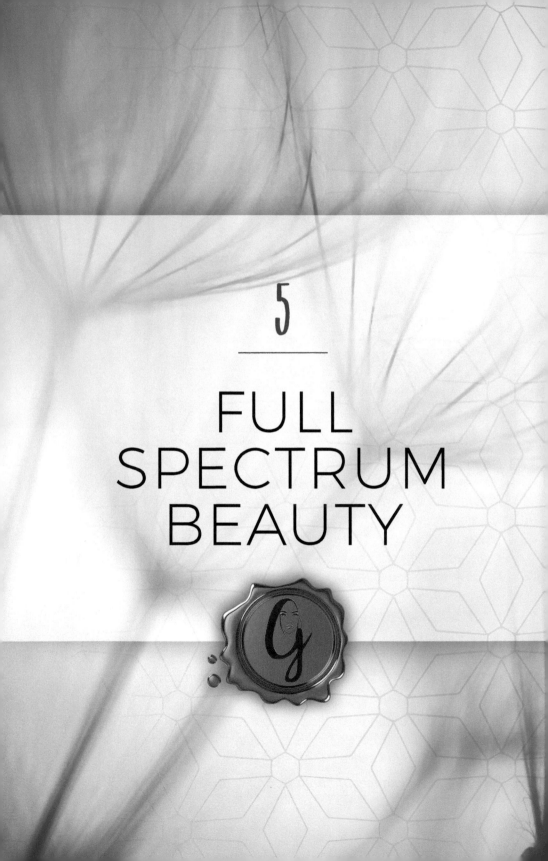

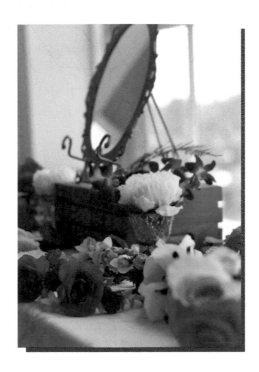

W

HEN WE HEAR THE WORD "BEAUTY," WE MAY TRANSLATE THAT TO MEAN SHALLOWNESS OR CONCEIT. We may need to pause, questioning our own relationship to this word. As women we have been made to feel wrong about being attractive. We've been told it's not safe and will cause too much attention. As a result we dim our light and "tone down" our playfulness with clothing and makeup. Some of us have even been tormented for being what others thought was "vain." In turn, we began to dim our light. And many goddesses were taught to equate their looks to their worth—creating false self-confidence. Never were we trained to discover our full range of majestic beauty. This chapter delves into the complete spectrum! It's an exploration of conscious beauty, intuitive beauty, spiritual beauty, and how to create beauty in your own home. Grab a glass of rose, kombucha, or green juice, and nuzzle into each word of this chapter!

Like most women, I had learned to focus on my outer beauty. I grew up in my friend's mother's hair salon in Detroit. I watched women sashay out the door with such an air of confidence, that I was sure you could smell it! Longing for some of that to rub off on me, I followed their lead. During my teenage years, I would spend hours getting cutting edge hairstyles and airbrushed nails that would stop traffic.

That would lead me to my very first career. Beginning my senior year of high school, I signed up for manicurist school. A few years later, I became one of the fiercest nail techs in Detroit. Outrageous nail-art, bold airbrush designs, and layers of rhinestones placed on top of long nails was what I became known for. It would be the same place where my passion for helping women was sparked. My clients and I would sit for hours talking, and it ended up feeling like much more of a healing session.

At 24, I was accepted to FIT to study fashion styling/marketing. I had this fabulous vision that I would be dressing A-list celebrities, shopping high end stores while picking up a little Gucci for myself, and of course traveling on private jets. I had a very *short-lived* stint with this! One day my professor sent me out to assist her on a styling job. Running from showroom to showroom, I found myself carrying enormous bags of clothing that kept piling on top of my tiny arms. This was a far cry from the glamorous life I thought I was signing up for. My dream was quickly shattered as my spirit whispered, "This is not for YOU." (My admiration and respect for stylists went up BIGTIME!)

As life would have it, I found myself signing up for a makeup class at MAC. It was time to add a little more glam into my life, now that I was living in the Big Apple!!! Totally inspired by the trainer who was leading the class and his stories of working with top models, traveling and being a creative mastermind, I decided I would try my hand out on my fashion designer boss right after class. Her daughter called me at 11p.m. that night, with such excitement in her voice, to tell me that her mother had never looked so beautiful! After that testimonial, I made up my mind that I was going to learn everything I could to be a TOP makeup artist.

I told myself that I had lots of experience with playing with colors and client relations, so makeup couldn't be that hard. For six years, a part of my dream was fulfilled, as I traveled the world working with celebrities like Molly Sims and Rihanna.

The glamor of it all wore off after a few years. Being on my feet for sometimes 16-hour days, mixed in with the toxicity of certain clients, was brutal to my body and blocking my feminine energy. By now I had been doing transformational work for three years, and it was becoming more of a part of my life. When I showed up as a "makeup artist" to these jobs, I feared that I had to hide that part of myself.

This was way before yoga and meditation ads were on the subway and spirituality became mainstream. There was something inside of me that was craving connection.

Up until now, my apartment was a place to rest my head and pay rent. I had done a little amateur decorating here and there, but for the most part, it was bare bones. I had never considered the idea that having a sense of beauty in your home feeds the feminine and supports the sacred energy. As I could feel the divine inner goddess blossoming inside of me I desired to bring candles, flowers and crystals into my home. I created a new website to represent this energy, and I shared chocolate and hand written notes. All of this was an expression of the beauty that was infused with desire.

One day I woke up in my apartment feeling claustrophobic. This happened to be *right* before I created my first Goddess On The Go experience. I could feel my body sending messages that it was ready to expand. After two weeks of going to look at overpriced, shitty apartments in NYC with several brokers, I felt defeated. I called my sister Ophira, who excitedly referred me to Feng Shui expert Katherine Mackinnon (www.creativefengshuinc.com). I was secretly resigned from believing that anything could change the dreadful feeling I had every time I opened the door to my apartment. Deep down I desired a home that I could love and welcome in my goddesses for legendary times together!

'PEACE OUT, BITCHES!' TO ANYTHING THAT WAS TAKING UP SPACE.

When Kate arrived, we began with a cleansing decluttering. Everything from pictures with exes to toxic cleaning products were chucked. "Peace out, bitches!" to anything that was taking up space. She suggested only bringing in items that brought me great pleasure to be with. When she left, my tiny one bedroom apartment felt spacious, welcoming, and energizing.

Within five days, I got out of a romantic relationship that I couldn't seem to shake, received an unexpected check for $10,000, and the creative energy juices were in overflow, with which I birthed Goddess On The Go. For two years this tiny apartment became my sanctuary of abundance and healing. When Will and I reconnected 12 years later, I knew this was a soul relationship. But my intuition said our romance

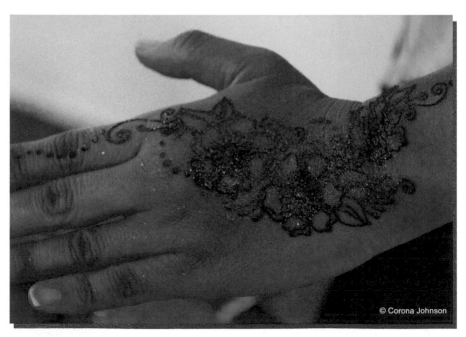

© Corona Johnson

was bound to fail if we didn't move out of this apartment and into a quieter location with more space.

I knew the first person I would be calling before we unpacked our boxes. "Feng Shui Kate" came over and did her magic. This time we set the intention of family, as I was welcoming in my honey and three bonus kids, who were becoming a part of my life. Three and a half weeks later, I discovered we had a new family member who would be joining us in nine months!

BEAUTY IS A HIGH VIBRATING ENERGY. IT CAN VISUALLY RETURN US BACK INTO OUR BODIES.

Beauty is like a wondrous playground and can make you feel as if you're dancing on a floor full of rose petals. It can return us back into our bodies and delight all our senses when we marinate in it. I'm thrilled to share my friends Tania Sterl, Britta Aragon, Monique Agress, and Dina Manzo to support you in taking your relationship with beauty higher! ✳

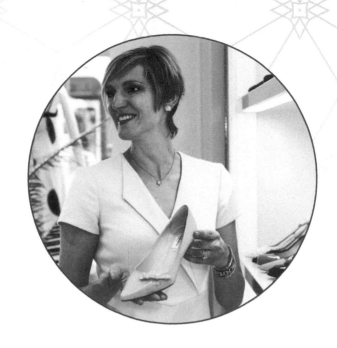

Beauty

WOMEN ON THE VERGE OF A BREAKTHROUGH

Divinely Contributed by

TANIA STERL

Introduction

WHEN YOU WALK INTO A ROOM FULL
OF WOMEN, YOU INSTANTLY SENSE THE
goddesses who wear their confidence for all to see. Tania Sterl was
that woman who caught my attention the first time I set eyes on her.
I can't pinpoint the words, but it was a strong knowingness—I had to
meet this bombshell sashaying about in bright red!

When we connected, I instantly felt a warm, down to earth energy
about her that made it easy to open up and share about our journeys.

Tania has bridged her sense of spirituality with decades of fashion
experience to support her clients in looking and feeling exquisite. She
has given me priceless style advice when I'm having moments of "Libra
indecisiveness." Tania always leads me back to my own truth around
my beauty.

Deep down, have you always wondered what colors bring out
your gorgeous eyes or what flatters your figure and makes heads do
a double take? Let Tania help you turn your fashion light ON! ✳

"

EMBRACE YOUR
UNIQUE VERSION
OF BEAUTY.
ACCEPTANCE
AND SELF—LOVE
ARE KEY TO
DRESSING AS THE
LEADING LADY
THAT YOU ARE.

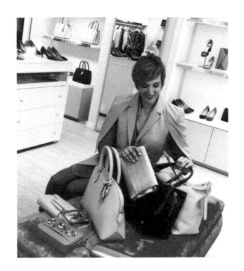

Q&A

WITH TANIA STERL

L: **Tania, we are just going to jump in and get intimate, are you up for that? Tell us a little something about yourself that most people don't know.**

T: Sometimes people's first impression of me is how model-esque I am with my tall, slender figure and angular features; they assume I must be in fashion. And they assume I look amazing all the time and it must come so easy for me! Once we converse, some admit they feel a little intimidated by me, and think that they have to be tall and thin to look good. But this is not true. To be truthful, my appearance and comfort in my own skin has been years in the making.

It comes easy to me now, at 45, as I've worked in the fashion industry for over 20 years. Yet I spent half my life not feeling beautiful. I looked like a boy when I was young. I was "underdeveloped" in high school. The "popular" girls had long, flowing hair, curvy bodies, were getting full breasts—and their periods. I was a skinny, shapeless twig with a figure more like a boy than a girl and short hair. In

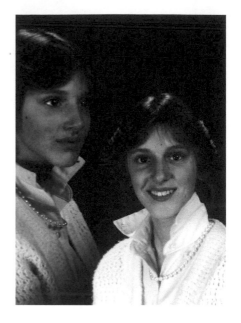

fact, I wore my brother's hand-me-downs and was made fun of for wearing "boys" jeans instead of Jordache. I felt like I didn't fit in. I was curious, I questioned things, I didn't like to follow.

I KEPT WHAT HAPPENED TO ME A SECRET—WHAT I CALL MY 'DARK, DIRTY SECRET.' ASHAMED, I BEGAN TO USE CLOTHING AS ARMOR, MY PROTECTION, MY DEFENSE. PICTURE THE TOTAL PUNK ROCKER.

I was bullied. I was called *faggot* and *freak*. The big boys who were older and stronger than me took advantage of this weak little odd bird, and would hold me against my will, accost me, and overpower me—leaving me feeling helpless and hopeless. I kept what happened to me a secret—what I call my "dark, dirty secret."

Ashamed, I began to use clothing as armor, my protection, my defense. Picture the total punk rocker. I shaved my head, dressed in black from head to toe, and wore spikes all over my clothing. I dressed to keep the bullies away from me. My favorite holiday was Halloween, so I could make two costumes and go out trick or treating twice. In disguise, there was a power in "hiding" behind my clothes, only later to realize, there's no such thing as becoming invisible. I had to face my fears, and be boldly myself despite the ridicule.

ONE'S STYLE CAN BE THE HIGHEST VISUAL EXPRESSION OF ONESELF, SHOWING OTHERS HOW BRIGHTLY YOU CAN SHINE, UNAFRAID, UNAPOLOGETIC.

A turning point in my self-acceptance was my junior year of high school. My literature teacher gave us an assignment to read an article and then explain how it related to each one of us. It was the 1990's so I wrote about my favorite supermodel, Linda Evangelista, who cut all her hair off and had a funny nose (like me!). A huge AHA hit me. I can be MY KIND of beautiful!

To this day I have short hair, my breasts are the same size as they were when I was 16—but who cares. It's my kind of beautiful and I work it! That's what inspired me to pursue fashion. To relentlessly express who I am inside and out through clothes, hair and makeup with no regrets. Even though I still wear black from time to time, I've softened; clothing is no longer my protective shield. I no longer dress offensively or defensively. I have the

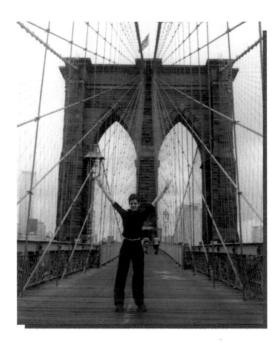

confidence to accept who and how I am with all my quirks. It's an expression of the vibrant, confident woman I am now inside and out, and I love to inspire others to do the same.

I'm happy to share with all of you how to dress your essence, embrace your beauty and be YOUR kind of beautiful, inside and out!

L: **"What do style and spirituality have in common that we do not tend to see on the surface?"**

T: To be spiritual is to tap into your "higher self" and to allow that "goddess" to be your guide. Whether you refer to that energy as goddess or truth or energy, do find time to connect with it. Try not to be ruled by the self that is self-critical or insecure or scared. Gently listen to that inner-voice for sure, then be open to the "goddess" who is kind, loving, accepting, peaceful, grounded, clear. One's style can be the highest visual expression of oneself, showing others how brightly you can shine, unafraid, unapologetic. Try to express the essence of your elevated self, that version of you inside that is composed, confident. Imagine

YOU to the 100th power . . . ! Honor where you are now, all the transformations you've been through to get here, and picture where you see yourself next, your future self—that's how to show the world how to behold YOU. By dressing as the leading lady of your life, you actually allow others to do the same, it's like giving yourself and others permission to feel and look that powerful.

. . . AN AFFORDABLE WAY TO PLAY WITH YOUR STYLE IS TO EXPERIMENT IN RESALE SHOPS.

L: **Why do we need to re-frame the way we view taking care of our outside selves as "superficial and frivolous" and not really mattering?**

T: Some consider style and fashion superficial or artificial, yet it's not. Consider this: Clothing is a necessity and part of our everyday self-care. It's interesting how many people put their clothing, their image *last*—it's the FIRST THING you cannot leave your house without, yet for most, it's the LAST THING they think about. Clothing is our second-skin, without it, that's like leaving a huge part of yourself behind. Bathing, grooming, make-up, and dressing up are primary parts of our daily ritual to honor our self-care as women. Think of women throughout history from belly dancers wearing gold jewelry to maidens braiding each other's hair; Ancient Egyptians lining their eyes with kohl. By honoring your self-value, adorning yourself with nice clothes, fun accessories, a hint of makeup, a beautiful hairstyle—it shows the world, "I'm worth it, I have value, I am beautiful, I care enough about myself to take care of myself."

Therefore, the two are intricately related: How you take care of your OUTER appearance is a reflection of your INNER well-being. Dress for YOU first. Make YOURSELF happy. That expression is different for everyone—you may have dreadlocks—you may be bare-headed or you may prefer no make-up because you're a farm girl, like my mom was! (Yet at Easter and Christmas she and my grandma would be all dressed up, hair and makeup done and all!)

Clothing and makeup should be used to make you look healthy and vibrant, and that's what matters. I encourage you to find a reason, an event, an occasion like a dance or a play date to dress up and dabble with a little make-up. Fashion and style are meant to be fun—so have fun exploring who you are inside and out!

SEEK OUT A STATEMENT PIECE LIKE A FUNKY JACKET OR A NECKLACE THAT FEELS LIKE YOU AND IS DIFFERENT FROM ANYTHING ELSE YOU'VE SEEN. IT'S NOT JUST HOW IT LOOKS. STYLE IS A FEELING. ASK YOURSELF, HOW DOES IT FEEL WHEN YOU TRY IT ON?

L: **What is one simple way a woman can begin her journey into finding her own sense of style?**

T: Start with your "fashion fantasy": Create a "My Style" Pinterest page, or get magazines and pull through them.

Find one hour to yourself. Pour yourself a hot chocolate or a favorite treat. As you page through magazines or browse online, don't think too much—just feel into what draws your eye. It could be a color, a texture, a print, an attitude, an overall theme. It could be a coat, a handbag, a shoe, a gem, or even a flower or animal. Then collect the tear-sheets and put them all on a vision board you can look at on your wall. Ask yourself: *What colors are you drawn to? What textures? What era? What feeling? Dark or light? 1920's flapper or 1970s disco doll? Soft or structured? Fur or feathers? Or a little dabble of both . . .?*

Then go into that closet of yours and pull out just five favorites that express that vision. If you pulled a 5" spiked leopard print stiletto out of a magazine—it doesn't literally mean you must have a pair in your closet! Try a leopard print clutch or a vintage pattern coat instead. Plus, an affordable way to play with your style is to experiment in resale shops.

Pick a power color you like then find something in that power color, like a peacock print scarf or a crimson cashmere wrap. Seek out a statement piece such as an embroidered funky jacket or a chunky beaded necklace or your grandmother's pearls. Play with something that may even have you thinking, "How dare I wear this . . .?" and is different from anything else you've seen. It's not just how it looks. Style is a feeling. Ask yourself: How does it feel when you try it on? If it feels right, or even a little scary, all the better—that's raising your style vibration!

... LET YOUR IMAGINATION RUN WILD! THIS IS YOUR 'FASHION FANTASY' TIME, SO THERE ARE NO LIMITS.

Beauty Ritual: Meshing Style with Spirituality

Step One: "I Love My Style" Vision Boarding
Start off by asking yourself a few questions:
Who are you now, and where do you picture yourself going next?
What is your #1 Personal Desire and #1 Professional Goal?

This is what I ask my clients before the shopping, before we dig in that closet. It's important to get clear with who you are, how you are, and what you are inspired to manifest next in your life, what events you need to dress for, and how dressing for them can help magnetize people and opportunities to get you there.

Next, create your "I LOVE MY STYLE" board:
Get a bunch of magazines. About 3-5. Fashion, travel, nature, health, fitness, etc.
• Don't think.
• Do this quickly.
• Pull what FEELS good. You may not even know why yet. Don't overanalyze.
• Trust the process.
• Fantasize!

Be sure to pull things that you almost hesitate on, or that have you silently say, "REALLY?" A huge emerald ring, a picture of Paris or India, a gorgeous pair of fierce shoes . . . two women on a beach, a man and a woman in the countryside, a woman by herself under a large tree, a fairy, a queen . . . let your imagination run wild! This is your "fashion fantasy" time, so there are no limits.

Once you have pulled everything, see if they fall into "categories"—shoes, purses, jewelry, coats, etc.

You may find also some *lifestyle categories* like romance, travel, places to live, nature, food, interior design—these all contain visual cues into your style preferences.

"INSIGHTFUL TIP": If there's something *missing*, like you pulled no jewelry, that could be a sign you may not see yourself as valuable. If you pulled more photos of water or far away places, maybe it's time for a vacation . . .! And you need a new swim suit or tunic for your trip. If that's the case, then consider collecting a meaningful piece of jewelry there, too, as your "travel treasure."

Be sure to glue down the ones you almost hesitate on—like, "OMG, I can *really* have that?!" Those are the ones to put on a poster board and post on your bedroom wall where you can see it everyday.

WHAT YOU DEVOTE ATTENTION TO WILL ALLOW IT TO COME TO FRUITION IN YOUR LIFE.

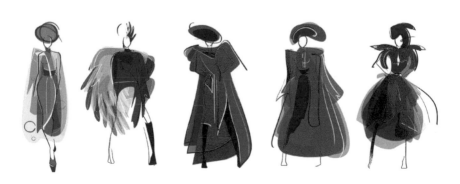

Now you have a map of colors to inspire you, dresses, pants, attitude, and it's time to come up with a NAME for your Signature Style. Will it be, "Modern Day Renaissance Woman"? "Exotic Woman Of The World"? "Classic Lady with a Vintage Twist"?

This way, when you shop, you only look for things that speak to your Signature Style.

Step Two: Breathe into Body Love Exercise

In order to dress that body, you've got to LOVE that body of yours! Flaunts, flaws and all. Even though there's no such thing as "flaws"— what makes you unique makes you memorable.

I once had a client go from a size 12 to 22 in five years due to an injury. She hated shopping. She was "too big" and nothing fit her like her skinny little friends. She swore she would never wear prints— too much attention. Well, by the end of our first personal shopping session, she was spinning around in a leopard print wrap dress exclaiming, "I'm gonna wear this on my next date!" So here's how to breathe in some body love . . . and dress all your beautiful parts!

Acceptance vs. Resistance Exercise

We can be so hard on ourselves when we look in the mirror. It is easy to point out the negative instead of what makes us unique and beautiful.

Do this right now: Make a fist, tighter, tighter, tighter, don't let go . . . not yet . . . tighter, tighter . . . hurts, right? Are your nails digging into your palm? What you are feeling is resistance. Does that feel good?

Now release it . . . ahhhhh . . . that's acceptance.

Which one feels better to you?

Create a supportive "opposite" beauty mantra:

RESISTANCE: "I hate my butt, it's too big."

ACCEPTANCE: "I love my rich derriere, and anyone worthy enough to be with me would be honored to get lost in my curves."

RESISTANCE: "My boobs developed when I was so young, I wish I could hide them."

ACCEPTANCE: "This is my goddess-given bosom. They attract attention. They are powerful. I own my power."

RESISTANCE: "My abdomen has never been the same since I had my baby. It's stretched and wrinkled."

ACCEPTANCE: "I am so grateful I was able to bear a child, some women cannot. What a gift!"

Breathe into those areas you love, and keep breathing into those areas you love not-so-much, until you've breathed into your whole body, heart and soul, with love.

ABOUT TANIA

Personal stylist for some of New York City's prominent female industry leaders in finance, fitness and media, Tania Sterl brings her 20+ years of fashion expertise to dress women for success.

Founder of Sterl on Style Image Consulting, her passion is dressing women through the important transitions in life—a change in one's body, age, relationships or career—and helps them dress with confidence throughout these changes, elevating their image and influence to the next level.

Visit Tania at: www.sterlonstyle.com and reach out for your very own personal style consultation.

You can also email Tania at tania@sterlonstyle.com. Get inspired by Tania's visual boards @sterlonstyle on Pinterest, Polyvore, Instagram and Facebook, too. ✳

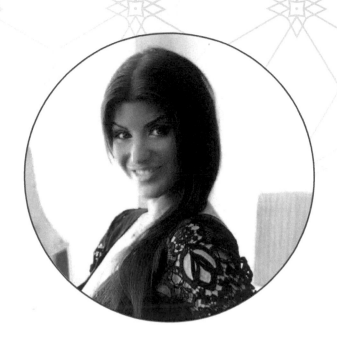

Beauty

PURA VIDA

Divinely Contributed by

BRITTA ARAGON

Introduction

YOU KNOW WHEN YOU JUMP ON A CALL FOR THE FIRST TIME WITH SOMEONE AND you can feel that you want this person to be in your life for a long time to come? This was Britta's and my connection. What was supposed to be a quick 15-minute convo turned into a two hour soul-baring talk! I knew a sisterhood had begun and I couldn't wait to meet her in person. What stood out to me was Britta's courageous story about her health. After being diagnosed with cancer and coming through it on the other side with her wellbeing intact, she stood by her father's side as he passed away from the disease. The average person would have crumbled from the grief and trauma. But what Britta did was use her father's death as angel fuel to create a clean/green skin care line that is free of those nasty toxins that caused the cancer they both developed.

Britta has turned extreme sadness into her life's calling—to serve and support people who are dealing with cancer and sensitive skin each day of their lives. She empowers people through her creation, CV Skinlabs, which is a kick ass skin care line that's totally free of any harmful products.

We pick up lotions every day, not knowing what is silently creeping around inside those bottles. Britta's daily mission is to help her clients find the resources and inspiration to continue moving forward in the midst of serious challenges, and she has created a sumptuous skin care ritual below, so we can deepen our level of self-care and rock out a goddess glow! ✳

I WANTED TO KEEP
MY FATHER ALIVE SOMEHOW.
THE BEST WAY I COULD FIGURE
HOW TO DO THAT WAS TO CREATE
SOMETHING IN HIS HONOR,
SOMETHING THAT WOULD
REFLECT HIS GREAT STRENGTH
AND INTEGRITY . . .

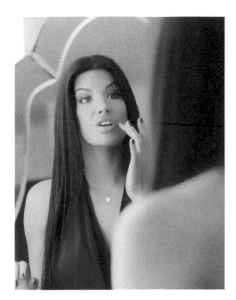

Q&A

WITH BRITTA ARAGON

L: **Your story is so moving, Britta. I have not lost a parent yet, and can only imagine that it must feel like losing a part of yourself, spiritually. Would you please share a little about how you found your inner calling shortly after your father's death?**

B: It wasn't easy. When we lose someone we're close to, it can feel like a part of us dies with them. I didn't want that to happen. I wanted to keep my father alive somehow. The best way I could figure how to do that was to create something in his honor, something that would reflect his great strength and integrity, and that would live on to benefit others, because that's always what he wanted to do—help others.

I ALSO PROVIDED INFORMATION ON NATURAL SOLUTIONS TO SIDE EFFECTS IN THE SKIN, HAIR, AND BODY, GIVING OTHERS ACCESS TO OPTIONS THAT MY FATHER AND I NEVER KNEW WE HAD.

The answer for how to do that came to me quite clearly. Both of us had gone through cancer, and had met many amazing people who shared that journey with us. I wanted to create something to give back to that community, and to make the journey easier for others who were going through it.

I used my background in health, nutrition and skin care, and combined it with what I had learned about toxins in everyday products, to create Cinco Vidas. That means "five lives" in Spanish—a nod to my father's battle with five recurrences of cancer—and the company became the foundation of everything that would follow. Through Cinco Vidas, I was able to raise awareness about the risks to our health present in the

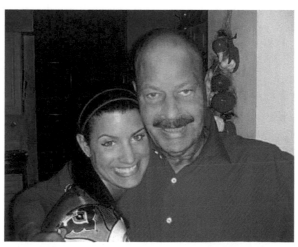

products we use on our bodies and in our homes every day. I also provided information on natural solutions to side effects in the skin, hair, and body, giving others access to options that my father and I never knew we had.

I also wanted to create something more, however. There was one experience during my father's battle that stuck with me. He was suffering from an acne rash, and I, being the skin care expert, got him a high-end cream that I thought would help. Unfortunately, it only made his skin worse, which was devastating to me.

That fueled my desire to find out what was really in these products that we were led to believe were good for us. Once I discovered many were full of harmful ingredients linked to skin irritation, allergic reactions, dermatitis, dryness, and even to health issues like asthma, diabetes and cancer, I vowed to create something different—something that, had it been available when my father was alive, would have actually helped him to look and feel better.

That desire led to CV Skinlabs, which is a line of skin care products full of natural and safe ingredients that are effective and nourishing. It can be used by anyone from those with medically treated skin to pregnant moms and babies, yet it is a favorite of fashion and celebrity makeup artists.

Through all of this work and dedication to the company and the products, I did what I wanted to do—I kept my father's legacy alive, and in doing that, came through his loss feeling like he is always with me, no matter what.

L: **Stepping into the world of green beauty can be a bit overwhelming, as there are SO many choices nowadays. What would you tell a goddess who wants to know why CV Skinlabs is in its own badass class, and why you are so in love with it? Personally, I do want to shout out a big song of gratitude to your "Rescue and Relief" spray—which saved me during my pregnancy, when I would wake up with the urge to ferociously itch my belly!**

B: What do I love about the products? Everything! (Ha!) But in answer to your question, I love that they are 100 percent safe but also extremely *effective*. So many times you have to trade. You get natural ingredients, for example, but the product doesn't work. It causes you to break out, or it doesn't moisturize for more than five minutes, or it doesn't soothe your redness, or whatever. Or, you get soft, moisturized skin, but meanwhile you're exposing yourself to synthetic fragrances, preservatives, formaldehyde, 1,4-dioxide, sulfates, and other potentially toxic ingredients that can cause skin and health problems.

With CV Skinlabs, you don't have to trade. You get both. You enjoy natural ingredients like shea butter, jojoba oil, vitamins, turmeric, oat extract, water lily, and many more chosen specifically for their nourishing and restorative effects, but you also get smooth, soft, radiant skin that gradually becomes healthier every time you use the products. You can see it! And I love that. I love that I can use something that I know is good for me, and see the beneficial effects when I look in the mirror. It's the best of both worlds.

WHAT THE SKIN REALLY NEEDS AT A VERY BASIC LEVEL IS A NATURAL MOISTURIZER THAT NOT ONLY HYDRATES, BUT PROTECTS FROM ENVIRONMENTAL ASSAULTS AND SOOTHES INFLAMMATION.

L: **For years I was clueless about where to begin when it came to taking care of my skin. Real talk here—I only started washing the makeup off my face at night when I was 33! Can you give us the skinny on "How to get that goddess glow"?**

B: Ha! Well, washing makeup off before bed IS key! But when we're talking basics, we absolutely must have clean skin. It has to start there. And so many of today's cleansers are just horrible, so you're right away causing problems like dryness and inflammation.

———————

Beauty Ritual: A fantastic (and simple) skin care regimen!

Cleanse.
Choose a safe, non-toxic cleanser that's free of fragrances and sulfates. Make sure your skin feels comfortable after using it. If it's dry and tight afterwards, that's not the right cleanser for you.

Moisturize.
What the skin really needs at a very basic level is a natural moisturizer that not only hydrates, but protects from environmental assaults and soothes inflammation.

So, in essence, you need a moisturizer that does three things: moisturize, protect, and soothe.

The skin is constantly losing moisture during the day as we're exposed to the sun, the climate, pollution, and more. Skin also loses its ability to hold onto moisture as we age. Dry skin is the source of damage, and leads to fine lines and wrinkles, as well as sagging and bagging, so moisture is critical, and not just the kind that sits on top of skin, but the kind that penetrates to get into the deeper layers.

PROTECT.

We need protection in the form of antioxidants, and we need to use sunscreen, too (zinc oxide is best), but a moisturizer without antioxidants is doing only half its job. Antioxidants help fight off free radical damage, and we're exposed to free radicals every day from the sun, pollution, stress, diet, and more. A moisturizer with antioxidants gives the skin the tools it needs to fight off free radical damage.

WE'RE LEARNING MORE AND MORE ABOUT INFLAMMATION THESE DAYS, AND WE NOW KNOW THAT IT'S ONE OF THE MAIN FACTORS BEHIND MOST SKIN CARE PROBLEMS . . .

SOOTHE.

Finally, we need something that soothes inflammation. We're learning more and more about inflammation these days, and we now know that it's one of the main factors behind most skin care problems,

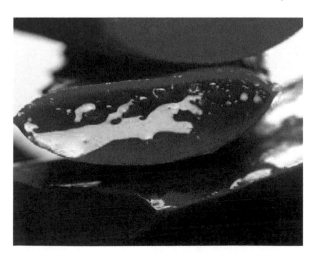

including acne, redness, rosacea, psoriasis, eczema, dryness, fine lines, wrinkles and aging. Your moisturizer needs to help calm the skin so that inflammation can't take hold.

(You can find all three in our products. Take our Calming Moisture, for example: It contains deeply penetrating triglycerides and has natural oils for moisturization, while ginger, turmeric, reishi mushroom, and other ingredients provide superior antioxidant protection. It also has oat extract, aloe vera, chamomile, and more, to tame and soothe inflammation.)

Just those three steps, if you choose carefully—cleansing, protecting and moisturizing—can help you enjoy healthy, radiant skin. That's where I'd recommend you start, goddesses!

ABOUT BRITTA

Britta Aragon, natural beauty and detox coach, author, and entrepreneur, discovered her passion for safe self-care while caring for her father during his eight-year battle with cancer. A survivor herself of Hodgkin's disease, she dedicated her work to her father's legacy.

She is the author of When Cancer Hits, founder of Detox Your Life Coaching and creator of CV Skinlabs, a safe, luxurious, and non-toxic skincare line that helps repair and soothe all types of sensitive skin. Britta's work has been featured in Organic Spa Magazine, People En Espanol, US Weekly, Telemundo 52, Real Simple Magazine, Fashion Magazine, Refinery 29 and more.

She raises awareness about safe self-care and the importance of reducing our toxic load physically, emotionally and spiritually through her speaking engagements, seminars, online workshops, private coaching and worldwide summits.

Visit Britta at: www.cvskinlabs.com ✳

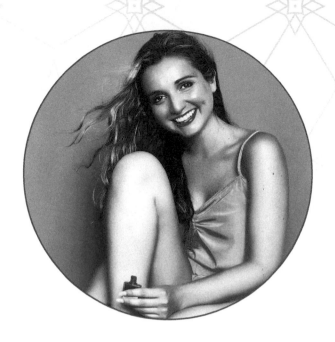

Beauty

CLEAN IS
BEAUTIFUL

Divinely Contributed by

MONIQUE AGRESS

Introduction

WELLNESS HAS BECOME A "THING," RIGHT, GODDESSES? WE ARE RUSHING TO GET OUR green juices and kale, but do we have the same urgency to clean up our beauty cabinets and makeup clutches? It may seem like another thing to do, but let me ask you: Isn't it worth avoiding hospital bills/ visits? Loving your body means ALL parts of it! Don't you worry, darlings, I'm not going to leave you researching for hours on end. One of my dear friends, Monique Agress, who I'm thrilled to introduce to you, has already done a lot of the heavy lifting for us! On her website, Goddess Huntress, she gives us the not-so-pretty scoop on what she calls "the dirty dozen"—namely, those ingredients we should be looking for (and avoiding like the plague) when we pick up that shiny pink lip gloss at the mall, or run to the nearest convenience store for an emergency tube of sunscreen on our way to the beach.

Monique's own journey in losing her dad to melanoma (skin cancer) was her motivation to help others get schooled on what we need to be aware of. For YOU, queen BOMBSHELLS, she created The Beauty Bag Toss Ritual, so we can get all up in your glam goodies and purge out anything that might be an ounce of harm to you. Deep breath, my loves: You are going to feel so much better by taking your health to a new level! ✳

INFORMATION AND OUR SPENDING ARE OUR SUPERPOWERS.

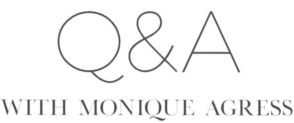

WITH MONIQUE AGRESS

———————

L: **Monique, I love how passionate you are about getting this knowledge out to women. At a time in the world when we have tons of online awareness around chemical-laden products, why do you think women still go for brands that may appear shiny and sexy but are full of toxins?**

M: Aside from being enhancers of our inner and outer beauty, beauty products boost happiness, confidence, and sensuality. So, when the topic of toxins lurking in your everyday beauty bag comes up, it is quite the beauty endorphin buzzkill. The idea of toxins in cosmetics does one of four things: intrigue women to find out more; overwhelm; make eyes glaze over in boredom; or shut down the information immediately and continue as usual.

We see the same reactions in the same regard to

controversial methods in the food industry. It is just human nature.

Luckily, women are taking the beauty buzzkill and whipping it into a successful buzzworthy beauty party. The clean beauty industry is a multi-billion dollar industry, growing at a rapid rate globally, and it is projected to grow like a weed to 13 billion in 2018. This is all because of the informed consumers!

Gone are the days of clunky, unrefined clean beauty products being sold at natural food stores. Now is the day of refined, beautifully designed, performance-formulated, clean beauty brands that attract both the informed and indifferent consumer alike. Large retailers like Sephora and Nordstrom have added clean cosmetics, skincare and nail color to their floors.

THE IDEA OF TOXINS IN COSMETICS DOES ONE OF FOUR THINGS: INTRIGUE WOMEN TO FIND OUT MORE; OVERWHELM; MAKE EYES GLAZE OVER IN BOREDOM; OR SHUT DOWN THE INFORMATION IMMEDIATELY AND CONTINUE AS USUAL.

Women are making large corporations like Revlon and Johnson & Johnson evolve, saying "no" to controversial ingredients just by using their wallets elsewhere. These large corporations are taking note and eliminating some toxic ingredients in order to gain back their market share. Information and our spending are our superpowers.

L: **What type of lifelong damage can happen to our bodies if we continue to use these products that the media keeps hush about?**

M: Unfortunately, there are ingredients that are carcinogenic, can cause respiratory problems, and manipulate our hormones. "Innocent until proven guilty" is not only the mantra for our judicial system, it is the same for scientific studies of cosmetic and personal care ingredients. Plus, the FDA is already spread so thin, proper and thorough regulation of the beauty industry cannot be expected, especially when they don't have full jurisdiction to do so. Crazy, I know.

GONE ARE THE DAYS OF CLUNKY, UNREFINED CLEAN BEAUTY PRODUCTS BEING SOLD AT NATURAL FOOD STORES.

L: **If you could write one thing in permanent lipstick on our makeup mirrors what would it be?**

M: My advice is just to stay away from the controversial ingredients now instead of waiting for a guilty verdict to do so. You will be waiting forever, and you shouldn't be a guinea pig.

YOU DON'T HAVE TO MEMORIZE INGREDIENTS, NOR DO YOU HAVE TO READ LABELS. SO MANY PEOPLE (LIKE MYSELF) HAVE DONE ALL THAT HARD WORK FOR YOU.

Tip No. 1:

Take a picture with your phone of this list to
keep on hand.*
Here are a few common toxic beauty product ingredients to stay
the hell away from—and why.

PARABENS (toxic to nervous and immune systems, skin irritant,
possible carcinogen)

SODIUM LAURYL SULFATE / SODIUM LAURETH SULFATE
(foaming agent, may cause hair loss, skin irritation,
may impair nervous system and cardiovascular function)

PHTHALATES (DBP and DEP) (endocrine disruptor, commonly
found in synthetic fragrance)

DIETHANOLAMINE (DEA) / TRIETHANOLAMINE
(TEA) / COCAMIDE (MEA) (carcinogen when crossed with
other ingredients)

TRICLOSAN (creates resistant bacteria, commonly found in
toothpaste and anti-bacterial soap)

RETINYL PALMITATE (potential carcinogen, skin irritant, commonly
found in sunscreen and anti-aging products)

OXYBENZONE (potential carcinogen, endocrine disruptor, common active ingredient in sunscreen)

TALC (highly potential ovarian carcinogen; tip: bring your own talc-free powder for bikini waxes and use talc-free powder on babies' bums!)

BHA AND BHT (toxic to immune, nervous and respiratory systems; endocrine disruptors; possible carcinogens)

HYDROQUINONE (possible carcinogen, may cause irreversible blue discolorations on skin and in urine, may cause arthritis, commonly found in skin lighteners)

TOLUENE (toxic to nervous and respiratory systems, found in nail polish)

PETROLATUM AND PETROLEUM BASED INGREDIENTS (endocrine disruptors, possible carcinogens)

(You can also go to Monique's website and view the list here: http://www.goddesshuntress.com/toxic/)

Tip No. 2:

Make this easy for yourself, not hard.

You don't have to memorize ingredients, nor do you have to read labels. So many people (like myself) have done all that hard work for you. Check out clean beauty blogs like Goddess Huntress, The Green Product Junkie, and GOOP to read reviews and learn about the latest and greatest products out there. Purchase beauty products from clean beauty retail sites like Beauty Counter, GOOP, Spirit Beauty Lounge, Saffron Rouge, and Honest Beauty, where they do all the nitty gritty label reading for you.

Go easy and have fun. There are some gorgeous brands out there that you are going to fall in love with. Your skin will show it.

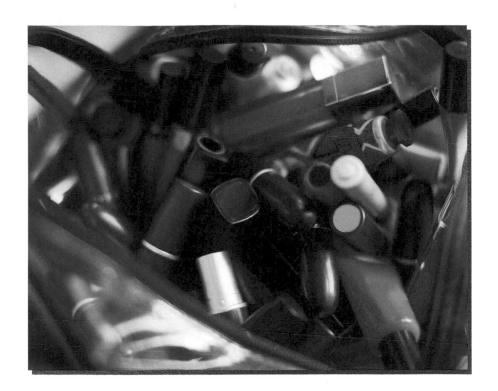

ABOUT MONIQUE

Monique lost her father to melanoma and took a stand to educate people about what goes into their products. Monique is one of the first clean beauty blog pioneers. She began Goddess Huntress with the interest of creating a bridge to connect clean beauty to glossy, mainstream beauty at a time when the two did not co-exist.

Now that the beauty market is abundant with a cornucopia of sexy, clean brands and very educated consumers, Monique is putting her focus into creating her new lifestyle blog—Boobs and a Babe, a place for cheeky mom anecdotes, family style, and family eats and wellness.

Visit Monique at: boobsandababe.com and goddesshuntress.com ✳

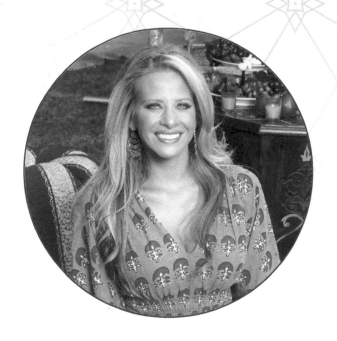

Beauty

ENERGETIC BEAUTY

Divinely Contributed by

DINA MANZO

Introduction

DINA AND I ORIGINALLY HAD THE PLEASURE OF MEETING AT A HAY HOUSE CONFERENCE several years ago. We shared an instant connection over her Pisces Sun sign and my Pisces moon—the love of having "no filter Sagittarians" in our lives, and gravitating towards all things woo-woo! One day on the way back from a movement class together, we were chatting about where I was feeling stuck. Dina shared some priceless insights about what I should get for my home to heal my heartbreak. I got rose quartz for each room in my apartment, along with a few other items she recommended, and things began to shift.

If you have ever had the chance to watch a past episode of *Dina's Party*, you know she is the B-O-M-B at blending opulence and spirituality, and if you have caught a past episode of *The Real Housewives of New Jersey,* you've seen glimpses of that famous altar she had in her closet.

We spend so much time in our homes, yet when our creative force is blocked, it feels as if we can't get SHIT done! My own space felt like that *forever*—and I had no clue that it was affecting everything else. It's so easy to let paper and things we no longer use take up precious space. I called on Dina for this section because I knew she was the Goddess who could help reinvent your living quarters!

Now, goddesses, I know it may be hard to part with your 10th grade Valentine cards, but TRUST me, you are making room here for what you really DESIRE! I suggest inviting a few sisters to support you in this energizing ritual. There is nothing like the feeling of walking into a home that infuses your pleasure and greatness! ✷

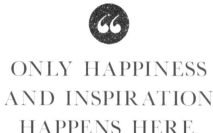

ONLY HAPPINESS
AND INSPIRATION
HAPPENS HERE.

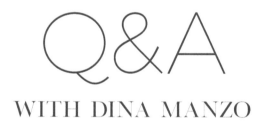

WITH DINA MANZO

L: **How do you feel your home affects the level of energy you are able to carry on a daily basis?**

D: Everything is energy. The place that you spend the most time should be filled with positive energy to absorb.

L: Okay Dina, beautifying our homes can seem mind-boggling right?! Often we are holding on to loads of "stuff" that carry a lot of charge from our past. What are the simple steps a Goddess On The Go can begin with?

D: I like to focus on the room you spend the most time in. Mine is my "lady cave"—my bedroom. For others it may be the kitchen or perhaps a spa-like bathroom. Other than filling that space with things that inspire you, I always suggest things that are fresh or alive. Fresh flowers, plants or it could be as simple as a crystal bowl filled with produce on your kitchen counter. Also getting rid of useless clutter—it declutters the mind.

L: Dina, I was so astounded at the things that started to open up and fall away when I began to reinvent my home to become my sanctuary. How can creating a space that you love affect your life?

D: Your home is the first thing you see in the morning and the last thing you see at night. It should be a beautiful, peaceful space to create amazing energy to take with you throughout the day, and to take with you into your dream state.

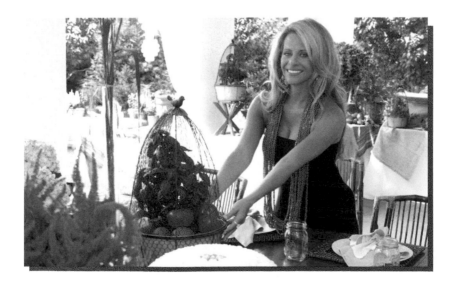

L: **What inspires you daily?**

D: The divine feminine energy that exists in every woman. Being in nature. Powers of nature make me choose a particular color of paint, or flower.

IT'S OKAY—YOUR AUNT WILL UNDERSTAND THAT YOU NO LONGER NEED HER DOLPHIN WINE OPENER FROM HER HONEYMOON.

Beauty Ritual: Energetically Clearing Your Home

STEP ONE: Identify the space in your home where you feel most inspired or to which you feel most connected.

Is it your bathroom, your bedroom, your kitchen? For me, it's my "lady cave" which is my bedroom and my closet.

Once you discover what that room is, take inventory: What no longer speaks to you? I'm talking about clutter. This takes up tons of physical and energetic space. Gift it, sell it, swap it, just say "bye bye" to what no longer serves you. (It's okay—your aunt will understand that you no longer need her dolphin wine opener from her honeymoon.)

STEP TWO: Smudge the cosmic sludge.

Once you have a clear physical space, you have to clear it energetically. I do that by smudging the entire area with white sage (you can use whatever you normally use to smudge).

STEP THREE: Fill the space with positive reinforcement and let all negative energy be gone.

Replace it with a positive affirmation: "Only happiness and inspiration happens here."

STEP FOUR: Introduce beauty to your space.

Now it's time to add in objects that give you peace and you feel connected to. A beautiful card, pictures of your favorite places or people in your life, crystals, stones, incense, statues, etc. You can set up an altar limlted to a corner of that space or scatter the items around. I do both. Personally, I'm drawn to the divine feminine energy, so I choose to place lots of Quan Yin and Mother Mary statues and beautiful images of both everywhere. But remember—this is *your* sacred space: There are no rules and no altar police coming to get you, so do what moves you!

Once you do this, you can keep it as your "spot" to mediate, pray, read, sing, dance—whatever it is that makes you feel alive and connected. You can also move on to other places in your home that you spend a lot of time in as well and do the same.

GIFT IT, SELL IT, SWAP IT, JUST
SAY 'BYE BYE' TO WHAT NO LONGER
SERVES YOU.

STEP FIVE: Reflect.

Take time to recognize what it is that you first see when you open your eyes in the morning and before you close them at night. What you see before you walk out your door … make those areas magical. (Yes, I'm talking about that cluttered nightstand.)

The purpose of all of this is to inspire and nurture your soul. When you look around, you have reminders of all the things that bring you peace and happiness. You will learn that you bring that energy with you throughout your day and, in turn, the rest of your life!

ABOUT DINA

Dina Manzo is an artist first and foremost...an artist, a curator of all things beautiful. You may have seen a glimpse of her passionate spiritual force on Bravo's Real Housewives franchise or HGTV's Dina's Party. Wherever you have seen her, its only a small window into her world of inspired living.

Currently residing in Malibu California she shares her secrets and products for living your best life on her latest endeavor: LivvTV.com

Visit Dina at: www.dinamanzo.com ✳

"

THERE ARE NO RULES AND NO ALTAR POLICE COMING TO GET YOU, SO DO WHAT MOVES YOU!

FINAL THOUGHTS

GODDESS MAGIC TO TAKE WITH YOU

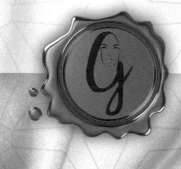

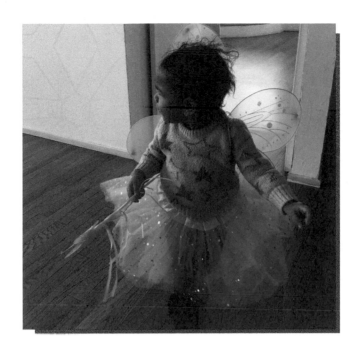

GODDESS MAGIC TO TAKE WITH YOU. Beautiful goddess sisters, as we come to a close, I am envisioning your spirit feeling FULL. That you remember your deep worth in the world and that you exercise it daily. I hold a vision that your belief in sisterhood has reawakened.

USE THIS BOOK when you feel doubt rearing its nasty head, or need some goddess juice to get you through an excruciating challenge. The exercises are designed to help get you to the other side.

This book is here to remind you that:
- Your powerful light radiates wherever you go.
- Your unapologetic inner badass is OK with exactly who you are.
- Your feminine energy is your strongest gift.

When the old disempowering stories come out to mess with your brilliance and pizazz, pull this book out and turn to any page. Trust that your divine intuition will lead you to where you need to be. To create the largest impact, apply the rituals of this book in sacred sisterhood, and create one if you cannot find one. Gift this book to another woman as a gentle reminder that she is seen and loved.

Please share any personal stories or shines that you experience on the blog or social media. I am eager to witness your bold rising of self-love and self-approval!

MY DREAM FOR ALL GODDESSES: Rise up alongside your mouthwatering dreams and desires, and allow the power of sisterhood to hold you through your deepest pains and highest celebrations.

xo,
Leora

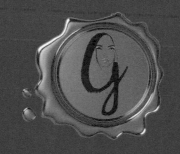

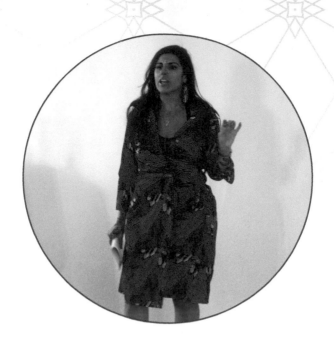

Final Thoughts

ABOUT THE
AUTHOR

✳

About Leora

HI, I'M LEORA! A proud, born-and-raised Detroit goddess! In 2002, I drove a U-Haul by myself to NYC where I found my second home.

I discovered **sisterhood** for the first time at age seven, when I joined the Girl Scouts. Around my teenage years, when you had to hide from your other friends the fact that you were still selling cookies and calendars, we disbanded and went our separate ways.

It was the first time I **experienced isolation**. No longer could I share with my closest girlfriends the abuse I was experiencing, the changes happening in my body, and the day to day challenges we all experience that often have us questioning our own judgment.

In the meantime, I tried everything to get that **exhilarating** feeling back! There was transformational work, eating healthy, becoming a creative being, and working out ferociously. But what I longed for during this process were the times I could gather with my girlfriends, listening to each other's stories with a deep understanding that only one woman can give to another. Nothing compared to the times with the girls where there was no agenda but to laugh for hours on end. It was a time we could drop our masks and be appreciated for every gorgeous layer we brought.

One day, I said enough of this **"being alone"** bullshit that society has forced onto women! The superwoman theory needed to be put in her grave. That week, I began a Goddess circle with seven other women who were craving sisterhood. This circle was a place where they could come and be seen and have a chance to express all of their emotions—from joy to sadness.

In our two years together, I saw tremendous growth! One woman no longer cared about the traditional standards of motherhood and adopted a child to fulfill her **dream** of becoming a mom, another left a job she no longer felt an ounce of happiness about, another travelled to places she had on her vision board, and all of us discovered our worth in our relationships and our bank accounts.

I couldn't DENY the powerful changes! It was time to bring this out to as **MANY** women as possible, and in 2012, Goddess On The Go was born. Goddess On The Go is a company that brings women together for one-of-a-kind experiences to rediscover that they ARE the lost treasure the world has been waiting for.

GODDESS ON THE GO IS A COMPANY THAT BRINGS WOMEN TOGETHER FOR ONE–OF–A–KIND EXPERIENCES TO REDISCOVER THAT THEY ARE THE LOST TREASURE THE WORLD HAS BEEN WAITING FOR.

Our experiences are designed so you will:
- begin to slow down and take exquisite care of yourself
- develop friendships with women that feel nurturing and safe
- find yourself taking risks which turn you on
- notice a richness that begins to affect all your relationships
- own your worth and begin to effortlessly make more money in your job or business
- have more FUN than you've had in a very LONG time!

Goddess On The Go has had the blessing of continuing to grow. Our events have been held internationally in Tulum, Mexico as well as in Hawaii, New York, Los Angeles and Detroit—and we are expanding virtually.

Our work has been featured in Elle Magazine, Lucky Magazine, The LA Times, and several others.

Leora Edut has spoken on stage with Marianne Williamson, been an expert on The Dr. Oz Show, and featured in the NY Post.

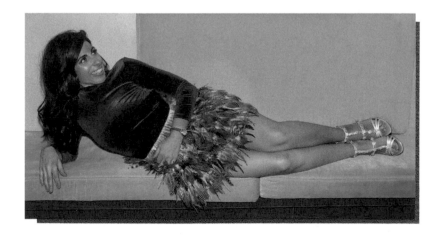

Testimonials

"I'm not sure if you'll receive this DM, but I just wanted to say thank you. I met you one time last year during group at GEMS. That one session we had was an eye opener. I learned from you that I was enough, and that I am a beautiful goddess. I took all the advice you gave to us in that group and I started loving myself more, and was able to get away from all the negativity around me. For that I'll always be thankful of you. I thought you should know the impact just one hour of me meeting you had on my life.

It's rare to find someone as inspiring as you, and I hope one day I'll be able to meet you again. I love your work. Again, thank you for opening my eyes. You're amazing and that's one trait you'll never be able to let go of."

—JENNIFER A.

"Hey Goddess of Beauty, just wanted to thank your energy for getting me out of my comfort zone and placing me in a space where I can expand the beauty of life. Had I never met you, I wouldn't have thought to have ever placed myself in a space with such a beautiful dynamic. And your presentation, truly captivating, bringing the very essence of what celebrating womanhood is. I came in stiff as hell but left out with a relaxed mood. Thank you for this introduction to self-discovery of my own womanhood. Love u dearly..."

—JACKIE C.